Simple Steps to Thin Thighs

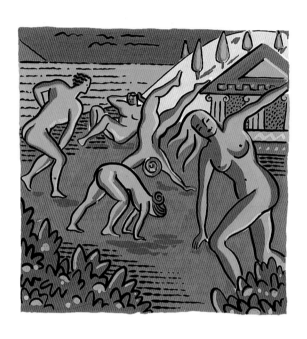

PHOTOGRAPHY: RICHARD TRUSCOTT
ILLUSTRATIONS: HILARY McMANUS

Simple Steps to Thin Thighs

Karen Burke, M.D., Ph.D.

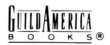

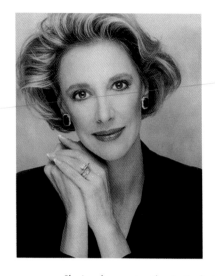

Dr. Karen Burke is a dermatologist and research scientist with a Ph.D. in biophysics from Cornell University and an M.D. from New York University. She is in private practice in New York City where she is also a Staff Member at Cabrini Medical Center.

Dr. Burke is known for her research on the prevention and reversal of aging of the skin as well as the prevention and treatment of skin cancer. She has also studied breast cancer and has published research papers on many subjects including fat structure and metabolism. She is a foremost authority in the field of cosmetic dermatology, and a frequent consultant to both pharmaceutical and cosmetic companies. Because she believes that "the best cosmetic of all is naturally healthy skin," she has researched and formulated her own exclusive line of Longévité® skin care products. Dr. Burke has written numerous articles and is frequently quoted as a health and skin care expert in magazines such as *Harper's Bazaar, Glamor, Elle* and *Family Circle*. She has made numerous television and radio appearances in the USA, Great Britain, France and Germany. She lives with her husband in New York.

Commissioning Editor: Sian Facer
Design: Martin Topping
Exececutive Art Editor: Keith Martin
Editor: Diana Vowles
Production Controller: Victoria Merrington
Art Director: Jacqui Small
Styling: Nato Welton
Hair and Make–up: Leslie Sayles

First published in Great Britain in 1995
by Hamlyn, an imprint of Reed Consumer Books Limited
Michelin House, 81 Fulham Road, London SW3 6RB
and Auckland, Melbourne, Singapore and Toronto

Text © 1995 Karen Burke
Photography, illustrations and design
© 1995 Reed International Books Limited

ISBN 1-56865-179-1

Printed in the United States of America

Contents

Foreword   6

1. "Beauty" and the female form   8
   The object of art is to give life a shape . . . . Jean Anouilh

2. Just what is cellulite?   14
   I've got you under my skin . . . . Cole Porter

3. The life cycle of cellulite   24
   It's never too late to be what you might have been . . . . George Eliot

4. Personal body analysis   32
   What lies behind us and what lies before us
   are tiny matters compared to what lies within us . . . . William Morrow

5. What your doctor can do   42
   The brightest seek the best advice. . . . P. G.

6. The battle for your brain   48
   The dream of change fuels the energy of action. . . . Edward de Bono

   Your personal cellulite reduction program   54
   A bad habit never disappears miraculously,
   it's an undo-it-yourself project . . . . Abigail Van Buren

7. Eat your way to a better you   56
   To lengthen thy Life, lessen thy Meals . . . . Benjamin Franklin

8. A better body in minutes a day   80
   Those who think they have not time for bodily exercise
   will sooner or later have to find time for problems . . . . Edward Stanley

9. Massage: from the skin, in   114
   Oh that this too, too solid flesh would melt . . . . William Shakespeare

10. Your cellulite reduction diary   120
    When patterns are broken, new worlds can emerge . . . . Tuli Kupferberg

Index   126

Recommended reading   128

Acknowledgements   128

Foreword

This is a book about a problem that affects 90 percent of women –
cellulite! As a physician, a scientist and a woman, I have enjoyed
the writing, and I hope that you will enjoy the reading. I dispel
misconceptions about cellulite and tell you what it is and why it
appears – and how you can reduce yours.

In the past, cellulite has generally been regarded by the medical
establishment as a superficial, cosmetic problem. But the psychological
consequences to a woman of even minimal cellulite can be taxing,
bombarded as we are today by advertisements featuring air-brushed
thighs, and the smooth, slim bodies of 12-year old girls who are
made-up and dressed as adults. Fortunately, medical research has
recently made great advances in understanding the causes of cellulite.
As a result, modern methods of treatment are now available to make
it very much easier for you to reduce cellulite effectively. This book
will teach you just a few new habits that can change your figure
without your having to alter your lifestyle.

No matter how out of shape you may feel right now, your body can
change within weeks – and starting to take control of your unwanted
fat instead of allowing it to control you will make you happier and
more optimistic. Your body is an amazing instrument that can respond
quickly to new conditioning and input. I can guarantee that if you
follow the simple rules I describe, after 30 days your thighs and even
your whole body will be noticeably sleeker.

There are questionnaires to help you pinpoint your motivations and
personal preferences as well as the ingrained psychological patterns
that shape your actions. By understanding these, you can almost

effortlessly replace self-defeating behavior with helpful habits. You will learn methods of eating to enhance your overall health and to reduce your cellulite, while eating delicious meals.

With my easy exercise program that takes just minutes each day, and concentrated sessions of 30 minutes four times each week, you will see your body change within just a few weeks. You will design your own special program that you enjoy, with secret exercises that you can do any time and any place. And you will learn methods of self-massage that reduce cellulite in minutes each day. Armed with these methods you will achieve and maintain a firmer, smoother, sleeker body while following your usual busy daily schedule.

It is with joy that I share the medical knowledge and techniques that will enable you to feel more confident, become more healthy, look more beautiful, and be a happier person. Let science work for you. And most of all, let's have fun!

NOTICE

It is always advisable to check with your doctor before beginning any diet or exercise program. If you have any medical condition for which you require a doctor's care or prescription medications, or if you have had injuries which might impair exercise, be sure to discuss your diet and exercise plan with your physician *before* beginning. Even if you have no medical problems that you know of, this might be a good time to have a medical examination. Please see Chapter 5 to learn how your doctor might help you lose your cellulite.

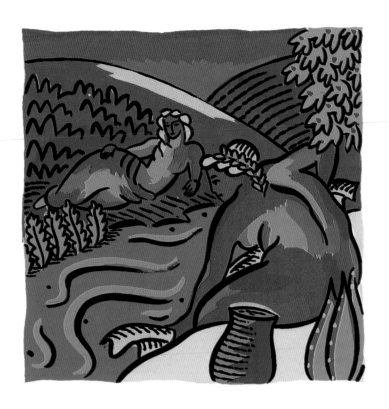

"Beauty" and the female form

Over the centuries, women's ample hips and thighs have been the subject of remarkable attention. In fact the cellulite-padded female figure found so unattractive today has been studied by anthropologists and also much celebrated by artists and historians, from ancient civilizations to modern times. Through the years, the perception of beauty has not been a static one. In earlier cultures, cellulite was admired; indeed there are very many examples of the artistic homage paid to this natural physical phenomenon. One of the oldest known sculptures (c. 20,000 B.C.), found in the Hypogeum of Malta, is a feminine form showing a copious stomach, large buttocks, and "thunder thighs," an ancient representation of femininity and fecundity. In Vienna's Museum of Natural History stands the ancient Venus of Willendorf (c. 30,000-15,000 B.C.). This primitively carved statuette, somewhat resembling a Pillsbury dough-girl who seems to be suffering from heatstroke, is less than flattering to today's image of the female gender, but she remains nevertheless an historic symbol of female fertility and pulchritude, a stone age sex symbol.

Prehistoric renderings of the female form, from the Mediterranean basin to the Scandinavian shores, emphasize the curve of the hips, thighs and buttocks. The figurines have minimal facial detail; the essence of the female was her pelvic roundness. Were these early artists drawing, painting and chiseling figuratively, or did they idealize their subjects? Did they see or only imagine and desire the abundant, pear-shaped female shapes they created?

Just as modern tastes change (for example from the more rounded, fuller feminine ideal of the 1950s to the more muscled and taut model of today), so body style evolved throughout history. By about 3,000 B.C., fat was out and thin was in.

The Egyptians idealized the smooth, svelte form. The thinner their bodies, the less clothes they wore. The upper classes strode the streets practically naked, delighting in the display of a well-toned figure. They expended great effort in oiling their bodies to moisturize their skin and to appear sleeker and better groomed. (The Egyptians were the first to use cosmetics as treatment to protect and rejuvenate their skin.) Ancient Egypt revered the thin female, as demonstrated by the elegant beauty of the Giza statue (c. 2,500 B.C.) entitled *Mycernius and his Queen*. No doubt about it: the Ancient Egyptians would definitely fit in at a modern-day department store!

The Cycladic culture of the Greek islands (c. 3000-2000 B.C.) is renowned for the simple, pure lines that are its artistic legacy. Its mysterious female figurines display slim, elongated forms. The *Callipygian Venus*, on the other hand, sculpted by the Greeks some 2,000 years ago, still forms an attractive model today, though she is far from slim. Her heavy thighs and buttocks, covered with cellulite, were considered by the men and women of her time as aesthetically beautiful. In fact, a free translation of this statue's title could be "Venus with the beautiful thighs." Throughout this period, the larger-sized woman was synonymous with femininity, fertility, good health, strength and survival.

The classical Greeks, known for the smooth, flowing lines so masterfully

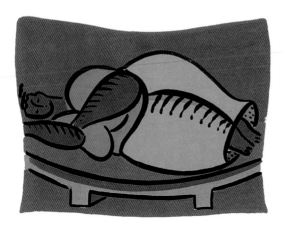

The prehistoric female of Malta; a buxom symbol of fertility and beauty.

demonstrated in their architecture, in due course chose to accentuate the lean, almost columnar figure of the female. *Kori and Dorian Peplos* (c. 530 B.C.) stands in Athens' Acropolis Museum displaying a svelte, block-like figure of a thin woman with a strongly accentuated waist. The simplicity of her garments form a distinct layer over her body, the fabric covering but not concealing her solidly rounded shapes beneath. Just as the treatment of her clothes is new, so is the form of her hair, naturally caressing her shoulders in soft, curly strands.

As the Roman empire flourished and grew fat, so did the Romans. Nudity was once again all the rage, and so the layers of cellulite sported by the women of the day were proudly revealed in Roman art. *Aphrodite of the Onidians* (c. 330 B.C.), majestically housed in the Vatican Museum, depicts a beautiful woman, thin from the neck to the waist; but the artist took his time to include plenty of adipose tissue below the waist, accentuating the abundant hips and thighs.

Christianity, with rising moral fervor, urged the artists of the day to cover their subjects so that flesh would not be sinfully exposed. (Perhaps this is why landscape art thrived during the tenth and eleventh centuries.) The wide vision of the Greeks and their students, the Romans, narrowed as the Church's crusades pressured artists to depict more austere and pious subjects. However, while portrait artists of this era painted women as thin, pale and fragile, it would be naive to suppose that dreaded cellulite had disappeared. It remained, but under wraps. Cellulite would not be seen again carved in stone or portrayed in oils until the Renaissance, the "Age of Light."

The celebrated Renaissance masters put paint to canvas, and once again the voluptuousness of womanhood was portrayed. Viewing Sandro Botticelli's *The Birth of Venus* (c. 1480) at Florence's Uffizi Gallery, you'll witness the beauty and grace of his Aphrodite emerging from the ocean, with seafoam at her feet, and cellulite on her arms, stomach and thighs. Isn't it comforting to know that the goddess of love had cellulite?

On the vault of the Sistine Chapel, Michelangelo emphasized the roundness of Eve's shape in his depiction of the *Fall of Man and the Expulsion from the Garden of Eden* (c. 1510). Poor Eve! Not only was she blamed for originating sin (a victim of bad press and poor judgment), but she was saddled with an inexperienced husband, evicted from Paradise, then had two ungrateful children and, according to the artist, cellulite! All this for eating an apple. We have here the first argument *against* the well-known phrase "the way to a man's heart is through his stomach."

In the Baroque style, Jean-Honoré Fragonard, obviously a fan of big women, painted *Women Bathing* (c. 1765). But no one honored the opulent female figure more than the famed Flemish artist Peter Paul Rubens. In the Louvre hangs his painting *Marie de' Medici Landing at Marseilles* (c. 1622-25). Although Marie de' Medici is the supposed slim-featured subject of the work, she is overshadowed by trumpeting pot-bellied angels who announce her arrival and beefy mermaids anxiously greeting her. Another of Rubens' highly acclaimed works, *Woman with the Mirror*, qualifies that subject as well for the comprehensive diet and exercise program presented in this book! Among other masters who notably represented the fuller-figured woman in their work were Leonardo da Vinci, Rembrandt, Raphael, Ingres, Watteau, Corot, Courbet and Renoir.

During the 1850s, the industrial age made it easier for women to mask their figure flaws. With the invention of the sewing machine, assembly line sweat shops flourished, and thanks to modern technology and the much improved transportation systems of the Victorian Age, ready-made garments – complete with form-fitted bodices, wide crinolines, and bustles – were made widely available. Complicated ornaments, detail work, laces, buttons and button-holes (mass produced by new technology) permitted a focus not on the body's actual build, but on the clothing styles and how women (and presumably men) wanted the female form to appear. Scarlett O'Hara's 18-inch (45 cm) waist was pinched by her tight corset while her voluminous petticoats emphasized the contrasting abundance of her hips and buttocks. Many women today might love to employ those tricks to hide a multitude of cellulite sins!

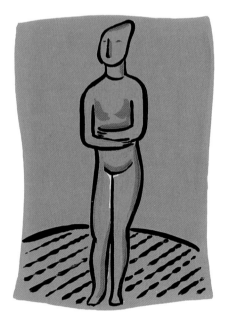

The Cycladic art of the Greek islands is renowned for its purity and elegance.

SIMPLE STEPS TO THIN THIGHS

Modern fashion technology made it possible for women to cover their fatty flaws, but they could not hide from the fact that cellulite survived. The fashion statement of the "gas lamp and speakeasy" era was a flat chest and a straight shape, but many flappers were buxom, as was the trend-setting dancer Isadora Duncan.

Throughout the 1930s, '40s and '50s, our female role models were voluptuously round. Betty Grable, the World War II poster sweetheart, sported seemingly cellulite-free backs of thighs. But I have my doubts. We never saw the fronts! And even Marilyn Monroe revealed the characteristic dimples of cellulite.

In the years following World War II American women were urged to be more full-bodied, round, voluptuous and sensual. After a tense time of rationing and lean-living and at a time when procreation was needed to repopulate a devastated world, the end of the war paved the way for those love handles. If a woman appeared well fed, she was considered well-bred. It was considered desirable during this time that "a woman look like a woman."

In modern art, the figure of the female form has changed. The women captured in oil paintings and water colors by Buffet or sculpted by Giacommetti no longer suffer from the rippling effects of cellulite. They appear to suffer instead from anorexia. Yet within the modern art movement the full female figure has not entirely disappeared,

as illustrated by the works of the sculptors Aristide Maillol and Henry Moore, not to mention the trademark roundness of Fernando Botero. Pablo Picasso, the most acclaimed artist of the moderns, depicted his women with the duplicity and panache of a seasoned politician; he magnificently covered the gamut of figure types from the svelte to the corpulent, incorporating his own sense of humor as he painted the fairer sex. The female form, whatever the shape, was at the center of Picasso's art.

The late '60s/early '70s ideal of the sophisticated woman, with ultra-slim hips and flat, almost boyish buttocks, was a creation of the fashion world, an ideal which might in part reflect women's growing desire, in some respects, to resemble men – an egalitarian, feminist ideal imposed on the female form. This modern-day body image – in tandem with the unisex craze – found its purest form in the fashion-passion for blue jeans. These work trousers, originally intended to be worn by men and cut with a rectilinear shape from the waist down, became and have remained a fashion must for women of the late 20th, soon-to-be 21st, century. Unfortunately, the ideal figure for these jeans belongs to the less than 5 percent of all women who, through heroic dieting and extreme genetic good-fortune, have the figures of men and no cellulite.

The 1980s through to the early '90s saw a further evolution of the ideal female physique. The lean and hungry look of the

'70s was replaced by the tight, muscular body of the '90s. This evolution not only accompanied the highly publicized and welcome trend towards the further empowerment of women, but also was given a very strong commercial push as "fitness" became a multi-billion-dollar industry, generating massive apparel and equipment sales, and causing fitness centers to sprout like mushrooms all over the world. The muscled look reached its apex with female body-building in which, at its most extreme, any hint of softness was considered a defect, and the entire concept of femininity was redefined in terms of a traditionally male norm.

Today we live in a commercial world that thrives on long legs and short attention spans. Advertising executives and their photography campaigns both reflect and determine our tastes, rather than our needs. Exaggeratedly stylistic advertisements barrage us with female models (many of whom are actually aged 12-20 but are cosmetically made-up to look 30), models who, as if by magic, have no cellulite, never did, and never will. If the dieting rigor of today's thin, young models were not enough of an imposition on today's female, there are the cosmetic photographic techniques of air-brushing the skin and elongating images to visually decrease the roundness of the female figure. Sadly, we in the real world cannot be air-brushed, nor can our figures be "touched up" by a master photographer!

So we continue to strive for the perfect body of today. A lean figure is considered by most to be the ideal, but in the real world, mother nature will not be dictated to by social whims. We may live in a "fat-bashing" society but nonetheless, cellulite certainly shapes our ends and, in time, can end our shapes!

In the merry-go-round of taste, we are in the process of broadening our vision, as we stand for the first time on the brink of a truly open, global society. Women today are becoming much more flexible in their concept of beauty. We are well aware of what looks are currently "in" and what forms are trendy. But we also know that we can recognize a good-looking body when we see one, regardless of trend, and that such bodies come in all shapes and sizes. Despite periodically exaggerated images of the ideal female form, influenced as such images are by art, photography, and advertising campaigns, history repeats itself: the natural roundness of the female figure is once again becoming more celebrated and appreciated.

Today, the most important aspect of beauty is health. The most admired female icons exude health, and any healthy woman has the radiance of beauty. This book is about your body's shape and your body's health. It is about doing away with our persistent enemy, the lumpy fat called cellulite. And it is about attaining and retaining a curvaceous, 100 percent female figure, to *your own* liking.

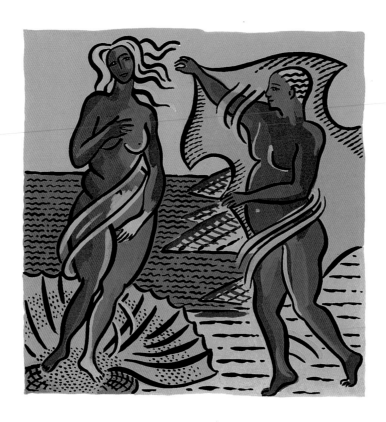

Just what is cellulite?

"Cel*lu*lite. *n*.: lumpy fat in the thighs, hips and buttocks of some women." *The New Merriam-Webster Dictionary*. If you want to win, know your enemy! In this chapter, I'll tell you all about cellulite – exactly what it is, and why it's in your body, where it is.

Mother Nature has quite a sense of humor: the anteater's snout, the chimpanzee's smile, or even your own experience at a 10 or 20-year reunion! Mother Nature might say to women, "Ladies, I've got good news and bad news. The good news is, cellulite isn't harmful to you; it won't make you sick. The bad news is, you're more or less stuck with it." I respond, "Without a great deal of effort it can be less, not more."

Cellulite is a natural female condition. Just as the development of breasts and the lack of body and facial hair are female gender characteristics, so is cellulite. Most women do have or will have cellulite. Several years ago the magazine *Marie Claire* reported that 95 percent of women over 16 years old admitted to having this condition in some form or other. In America, scores of surveys demonstrate how much we care about our cellulite, which is usually deposited on the buttocks, hips, and thighs, and sometimes on the lower part of the abdomen and the upper arms. Every woman can develop these fatty deposits, but every woman can also improve her condition, and that's what this book is all about!

Cellulite is not a disease. Cellulite is neither "trapped toxins," nor "internal pollution," nor "inflammation of cells." It is a natural characteristic of the female body, plain and simple.

Some doctors tell us that cellulite does not exist. In fact, 14 years ago, the *Journal of the American Medical Association* stated, "There is no medical condition known or described as cellulite." (Right, and the earth is flat!) The controversy is not about the actual condition, but about the word itself. It was first coined in 1816 by Dr. W. Balfour, who contributed the term to French medical literature. (The earliest definition of cellulite appeared in French dictionaries before 1900.) The French term has often been mistranslated in English to *cellulitis*, which means "an inflammation or infection of cells," but the specific cause of cellulite, as you will learn below, does not involve any such inflammation or infection. Although the alternative name *lipodystropy* (literally, "defective nutrition of fat") does not convey a true description of the problem, this term has been proposed as a means of resolving the debate in the medical and lay press. In fact, a number of medical experts and doctors have suggested more accurate and descriptive terminology. I'm sure you will agree, however, that names such as *dermo-panniculosis deformans* ("deformed skirt of skin tissue"), *status protrusis cutis* ("state of protruding skin"), or Dr. Stockman's 1904 proposal, *panniculosis adiposus* ("extra skin tissue around fat") are not exactly catchy. Imagine hearing a friend lament the "*dermo-panniculosis deformans*" on her thighs!

I vote that we retain the French word "cellulite," recognizing its meaning as the distinct distribution of fat in the female lower body with the dimpling of overlying skin. The term today is a popularly recognized and accepted one, used by the many women who share the condition.

WHY DOES CELLULITE LOOK DIFFERENT THAN OTHER FAT?

When a young girl reaches puberty, female sexual hormones, especially estrogen, cause her to develop breasts, hips, and the typical curves of the female form. Estrogen also induces the enhancement of fat on the lower body, especially on the thighs and hips. (By contrast the male hormone, testosterone, induces fat loss in those areas along with some fat enhancement in the deltoids and chest.) When the female fat cells enlarge in response to increased estrogen, the door is wide open for cellulite to appear! If and when the condition becomes noticeable, it takes on the appearance (regrettably!) of a fleshy orange peel or a lumpy mattress.

Do you have cellulite? Try the dreaded "pinch test" (see the diagram on page 19). Just squeeze about 4 inches (10 cm) of skin on your lower, inner thigh horizontally between your fingers. Don't be alarmed if one of the two types of cellulite makes its appearance. If your skin resembles citrus rind, you have the world-renowned "orange peel phenomenon." If you see an alternating pattern of fat protrusions and linear depressions, that's the "mattress phenomenon." The lumpier the cellulite (or more mattress-like its appearance) the more fat is stored. The condition is aptly named: many women, on discovering these lumps on their thighs and buttocks, have wanted to take to their mattresses and hide!

Both the dimpled look and the lumpy ripples are caused by the way the fat is anchored beneath the skin and by the way this fat is stored in fat cell compartments surrounded by thickened dividers of connective tissue. Remember, the fat stored in our bodies is not firm or solid: it ripples because it is softer and more spongy in texture than other tissue such as skin or muscle.

THE IMPORTANCE OF FAT

The average woman has 20 to 60 *billion* fat cells (a depressing thought!). Although you might have thought that fat is found only under the skin, it is actually stored throughout the body, within bone marrow, between muscle fibers, and around all of the internal organs. In fact, believe it or not, the only places in the human body free of fat are the eyelids, the scalp, the earlobes, the palms of the hands and soles of the feet, the labia, the penis and the scrotum. Pinch the skin on your palm; it is tight and firm precisely because there is no deposit of fat underneath. This is pure skin with connective tissue.

The layer of fat just under your skin is important to you both mechanically and metabolically. It forms a cushion, protecting your body against external pressure and acting as elastic padding between your skin and the deeper layers of muscle underneath – your shock absorber, so to speak. In the fat cell's defense, let it be said that fat cells are a necessity for our

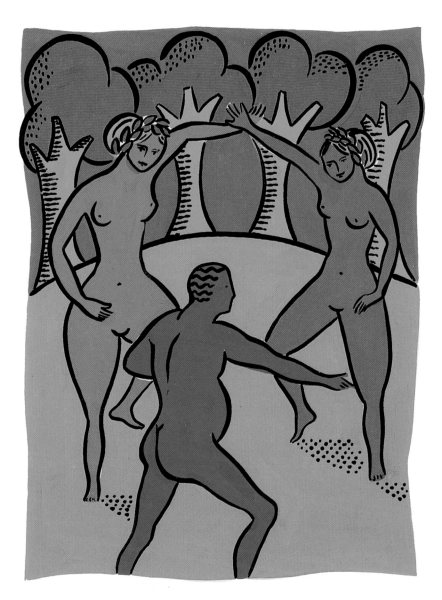

Apples and pears: why do women accumulate excess fat on different parts of their bodies to men?

survival. Prehistoric humans weren't raised on three nutritionally balanced meals a day; on the contrary, our species was generally closer to starvation. Fat served then, as now, as the storehouse of our energy and the mechanism for keeping our body warm.

Don't think of your fat cells (or adipocytes) as merely absorbing fat and

17

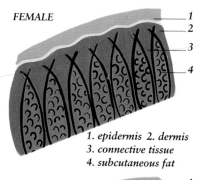

FEMALE

1. epidermis 2. dermis
3. connective tissue
4. subcutaneous fat

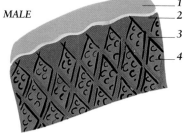

MALE

The structure of a woman's skin and connective tissue, as compared to a man's, causes the appearance of cellulite.

hanging onto it forever. Your fat cells metabolize, or process, fat and then release part of this deposited fat in the form of molecules called lipids (we commonly call this substance fat). Your fat reserves are not static; they are dynamic, continuously forming and degrading lipids, alternately storing energy from dietary nutrients in your fat cells, then breaking down that fat to release the energy which is essential for all your bodily functions.

THE STRUCTURE OF CELLULITE

In 1978, Doctors Nuremberger and Muller led a Berlin research team to clarify the precise structure of cellulite. For more than eight years they studied the structure of female and male skin and tissue under the skin (the subcutaneous or so-called deep fat), analyzing 180 tissue samples. Their findings clarified a great deal: Nuremberger and Muller observed a very distinct difference between female and male in the structure of the connective tissue that surrounds, or "packages" fat cells under the skin of the thighs. Specifically, they noted differences in the form of the dividers (the septa) which package fat cells.

In women, the doctors discovered, fat cells are grouped within sacs, divided by connective tissue arranged in a vertically-arched design attached to the deep layer (the dermis) of overlying skin to form "standing fat cell chambers." From these fat cell chambers, little anchors project upwards into the lower layer of the skin, dividing the regions of the deep dermis, with their surrounding glands and blood vessels. Under pressure, these vertical fat cell chambers change shape more than volume, their vertical protrusion becoming more evident at the skin's surface. The result – the appearance of lumpy cellulite! When a sack of tomatoes is pressed tightly, the surface appears lumpy. In the same way, if fat cells inside the connective tissue sacs enlarge, as they do when you gain weight, they force the skin to stretch tightly across the fat, making your thighs look dimply.

However, in the comparable skin of men's thighs, the connective tissue anchors are structured in a more horizontal honeycomb or lattice-like pattern, packaging fat cells in small polygonal units. The connective fibers in males are not only more numerous, but tend to

18

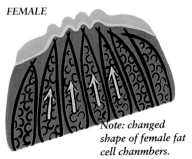

FEMALE

Note: changed shape of female fat cell chanmbers.

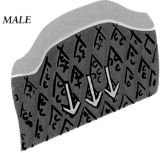

MALE

A simple "pinch test" reveals the dimpling, or orange peel effect, of cellulite on a woman's thigh, but not on a man's.

penetrate at an angle (as opposed to straight up and down for women) like the strings of a parachute. Because of this net-like architecture, as male fat cells enlarge, they do not protrude straight into the dermal layer of the skin, and they do not therefore cause corresponding rippling on the skin's surface. The outer layer of a man's skin is thicker than a woman's, further insulating the male from surface lumpiness. To top it all off, the packages of fat in women are larger than in men (for example, the size of grapes versus the size of blueberries). Needless to say, a plastic bag full of grapes looks lumpier than a cloth sack full of blueberries!

Drs. Nuremberger and Muller demonstrated that this packaging of fat cells is hormonally determined. In the development of a fetus, the characteristics of the male become evident only as of the sixth or seventh month, at which time the male hormones are first formed. Only then, just before the actual birth, does the structure of the packaging of fat cells in the male change so that he will not later develop cellulite. Before that, his fat cell structure is just like a female's.

These differences in male and female surface and sub-surface tissue become accentuated with age.

As we women grow older, our connective tissue anchors thicken while our surface skin becomes thinner and less elastic. As a result, our skin is less resistant to pressure coming from bulging fat chambers beneath. More rippling can appear, and the dimpling of cellulite can be exaggerated. Pressure from the fat under our skin's surface can also cause stretching, giving our hips, thighs and buttocks the additionally unattractive appearance of enlarged pores, the "orange peel phenomenon" or *"peau d'orange"*.

Like it or not, women are by nature susceptible to cellulite. There are no differences between the actual fat cells that can be found in women or men; the differences are in the texture and structure of the subcutaneous packaging of those cells, with regrettable consequences for the female of the species!

THE INFLUENCE OF HORMONES

If you're really interested in controlling those fat cells, you should learn how normal fat cells grow. A person is born with a certain number of fat cells (or adipocytes) determined by ethnic and genetic factors. The number of these fat cells increases until the age of two, depending upon the initial diet of the infant. The only other times that the *number* of fat cells increases are during puberty, or with a major weight gain leading to obesity.

During puberty the male hormone testosterone causes these effects on connective tissue:

1. Enlargement of all the muscles.
2. A decrease in the size of fat cells in the lower part of the body, as in the male hips and thighs.
3. An enlargement of the size of fat cells in the shoulders and upper chest.

The female hormone estrogen has a different effect:

1. No enlargement of the muscles.
2. No enlargement of the size of fat cells in the shoulders.
3. An increase in the size of fat cells below the umbilicus, particularly on the hips, buttocks and thighs. In some cases this increase may even extend as far as the knees.

Because of the female's hormonal influences, a normal woman has more fat cells than a man. In fact, an average woman of 21 has almost *twice* the volume of fat as a man of the same age. Women have on average about 22 percent body fat, while men have only 12 percent. It's simply not fair!

As we learned, not only does estrogen cause the localization of more and larger fat cells on the lower part of the female body, it also makes the skin's dermis layer thinner so those underlying fat cell packages are more apparent on the skin surface. Men's testosterone gives the added advantage of thicker body hair which "buttresses" the thicker skin, lessening further the appearance of surface rippling.

Finally, estrogen causes some retention of water, unlike testosterone which does not. As a result, during the important phases of a woman's life when hormonal levels are increased, especially during puberty or with the ingestion of oral contraceptives, there can often be an apparent increase in cellulite.

The effect of hormones on the structure of the skin and its subcutaneous tissue is particularly noticeable in men with a rare genetic disease called Kleinfelder's Syndrome. Men afflicted with this disease have an extra female X chromosome – i.e. a chromosome structure of XXY. (X is female and Y is male. Normally, women have the chromosomes XX and men have XY.) Drs. Nuremberger and Muller showed that those patients with such a severe androgen deficiency demonstrated a female pattern of connective tissue and a female type of fat distribution in the thigh and hip region with a positive dimple phenomenon. The researchers did not find the dimpling phenomenon in any men with normal levels of androgens, whether or not they were overweight. Men who are treated with female hormones do take on some physical feminine traits, including cellulite, just as women who are treated with male hormones lose weight from their hips and thighs and deposit it on their stomachs. All this adds up to one conclusion: it is clear beyond doubt that the presence of cellulite is primarily induced by female hormones influencing connective tissue and fat cells.

APPLES AND PEARS

We all know the sad fact that when women become overweight, their excess is mainly on the thighs and buttocks; women become pear-shaped. Men, on the other hand, become apple-shaped, with their excess in the belly. This distribution is caused not only by hormones, but also by the enzyme lipoprotein lipase on the fat cell surface which transports fat into the cell. The greater the activity of this enzyme, the more fat taken is taken in. Genetically heavier individuals have increased enzyme activity. In women, the lipoprotein lipase activity is higher in the thighs and buttocks, and in men the activity is higher in the visceral fat cells of the abdomen. When we eat too much, these specific cells soak up the fat like a sponge, giving us these unflattering shapes.

BLOOD VESSELS

There's more to the story. When a woman becomes overweight, other negative factors come into play: fat cells enlarging within each sac of connective tissue with time cause double trouble – reduced blood flow and reduced drainage of the lymphatic system. (In other words, when you gain weight, you're really gumming up your body's hydraulic system!) Studies done by Dr. Sergio Curri in Milan show that there exists fine-tuned regulation of blood flow within your fat tissue. Using electron microscopy, Dr. Curri discovered blocking devices in the tiny blood vessels that supply the fat cells. These devices act as little valves controlling the flow of blood.

If the fat cells enlarge, pressure on the micro-blood vessels causes these little valves to constrict blood flow. To put it simply, when we gain weight, our circulatory system will not function to its proper standard, further contributing to the appearance of cellulite!

FAT TRANSPORT, STORAGE AND METABOLISM

Here's one final piece to the puzzle. The way our body processes (metabolizes) fat is a dynamic process.

This is how it works:
1. We absorb dietary fat from the intestines;
2. We both store and synthesize fat (as lipid molecules) in the liver;
3. We transport this dietary fat and synthesized lipid as triglycerides in our bloodstream to the fat cell;
4. The enzyme lipoprotein lipase on the surface of the cell breaks down the

triglycerides into glycerol and free fatty acids to allow fat to enter the fat cell;

5. Triglycerides are re-formed within our fat cells for storage of fat;

6. When we need energy, the store of triglycerides within our fat cells is again broken down and the free fatty acids are moved out to fuel muscles.

The synthesis and the storage of fats is governed by genetic, hormonal and biochemical factors. Certain female hormones such as prolactin, oxytocin, and estrogen, as well as growth hormone, stimulate the synthesis of fats in the liver.

The breakdown of fats (lipolysis) is controlled by many factors, especially by hormones such as adrenaline, glucagon, noradrenalin, thyroid stimulating hormone, melanocyte stimulating hormone and adrenal corticoptropic hormone (ACTH). Other hormones act more slowly to increase lipolysis: these include glucocorticoids and growth hormones which act on the synthesis of the fat enzymes. Hormones such as pituitary hormones, thyroid hormone and adrenaline also facilitate lipolysis. The nervous system further aids lipolysis, not only regulating the output of hormones, but also acting directly upon the so-called adrenergic receptors on the actual membrane of the fat cell.

Certain foods and medicines can alter lipolysis. For example, caffeine, as well as certain medicines such as theophyllin and aminophylin (which is frequently used to treat asthma), can increase the breakdown of fat. This point is important because many new anti-cellulite creams which contain these compounds are now available on the market.

Eating foods which are too rich in fats and eating too much, especially after a fast, activates the movement of fat into the fat cell. The activity of lipoprotein lipase is increased with the release of insulin (stimulated by eating sugar), permitting more fat to be transported into the fat cell. Conversely, the enzyme's activity is decreased with fasting, after strenuous muscular exercise, and with lack of insulin (such as in diabetes). Now you're beginning to get the picture! As you exercise and control your eating, you are actually reducing your body's production of the enzyme that moves fat into your fat cells. Need I say more?

SUMMARY

Cellulite is caused by the fact that the connective tissue sacs surrounding women's fat cells are arranged in a vertically arched pattern, attaching directly to the underlayer of the skin (rather than the net-like pattern found in males).

As a result of the influence of female hormones and the natural aging process, a woman's skin becomes thinner and the fat cells in the areas of her stomach, thighs and buttocks become larger. This enlargement of fat cells within the limiting sacs of connective tissue makes surface

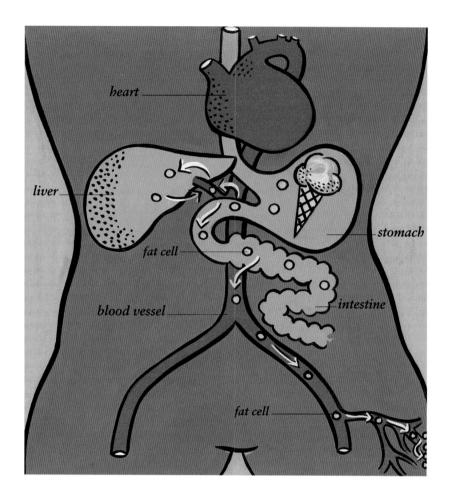

The fat you eat is absorbed from your intestine and transported through your blood, either directly or via your liver, to your fat cells.

dimpling more evident. In response to female hormones or weight gain, the enlargement of fat cells also causes alterations in small blood vessels, sometimes even resulting in slower blood flow. All of these effects are cumulative in the overweight or obese individual, and each of these changes aggravates the others. The result is a cycle of progressively worsening cellulite – unless and until that cycle is ended.

That's what this book is about. If you follow my *Simple Steps to Thin Thighs* plan which you will find outlined on pages 54-55, you will retard the process of worsening cellulite and, hopefully, bring it to a halt. You may even succeed in eliminating the appearance of cellulite altogether!

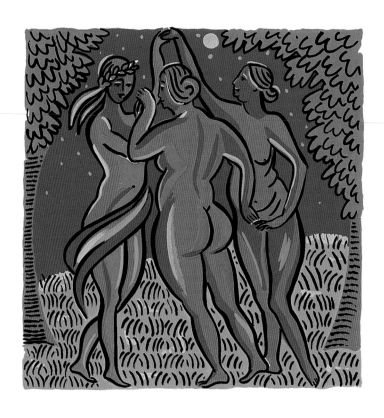

The lifecycle
of cellulite

Our "womanish figure" comes from our hormones acting as designed – but hormones sometimes take a bad rap, blamed as they are for rampant emotions, abnormal behavior and cellulite – an "excess of femininity." By understanding the natural development of cellulite during the important phases of a woman's life, we can help protect ourselves from this excess we can well do without!

PUBERTY

Philosophically, puberty is a time when we stop asking questions and begin questioning answers. Physiologically, puberty is the most difficult time in an adolescent's life. The anxieties, agonies and psychological pressures resulting from the hormonal changes that occur during the teenage years should be neither neglected nor rejected.

At puberty, girls become sensitive about their physical development. Suddenly that flat chest needs a bra. For some girls, sensitivity about breast development can be not only embarrassing, but agonizing. And we can all recall the sudden appearance of a pimple – the threat of acne – foreboding possible catastrophe on the night of a big date. Added to these psychological traumas, a girl begins to menstruate – all of these physical changes happening seemingly overnight. To top it all off, she begins to develop cellulite!

Many experts believe that reproduction is dependent upon body fat to encourage estrogen secretion. At puberty, estrogen is secreted by our ovaries for the first time, with consequent effects upon our bodies. Estrogen increases fat in the hips and thighs, the so-called "saddle-bags" or "*culotte de cheval*", sometimes as far down as the knees – the "jodhpur look." The percentage of fat in the female body goes from roughly 15 percent at the age of 15 to 22 percent at the age of 21. (And that's for those women who are *not* overweight.)

Estrogen can sometimes affect our appetites, especially during puberty. Do you remember a couple of days each month when you felt absolutely ravenous for something greasy or sweet, for foods, or combinations of foods, you wouldn't normally have eaten?

A girl in the throes of puberty may also begin to retain water, contributing to the appearance of cellulite. Water retention can be more severe in girls who suffer from pre-menstrual syndrome (P.M.S.), which is a particular problem in our puberty and post-puberty years. There's a special reason for this. During this time, a young girl has many anovulatory cycles (in which no egg is released), resulting in an imbalance in the estrogen-progesterone ratio during the second phase of the menstrual cycle. Excessive water retention is due not only to higher levels of estrogen, but also to low levels of progesterone, the hormone that usually counterbalances the water-retentive activity of estrogen in a young girl.

With occasional increase in the number of fat cells and with the enlargement of each cell compounded by water retention, the fat cells packaged in connective tissue sacs (described in Chapter 2) cause pressure on the blood vessels, weakening normal endarteriolar blocking devices, in due course initiating a gradual thickening of capillary walls in cellulitic areas. It is important to note that if indeed changes occur to the blood vessels, they are a consequence of the initial presence of cellulite and not its cause. But if these blood vessels actually do change, it does become more difficult to combat cellulite.

What happens to water retained during and prior to menstruation? In the deeper layer of the skin, between the cells, are proteoglycans – most prevalently hyaluronic acid, a molecule always thirsty for water. In fact, hyaluronic acid can retain from 6 to 1800 times its weight in water (the average being about 300 times its weight)! As the hyaluronic acids retain more and more water, they organize into longer and longer chains. This results in your body's storing more water and retaining it longer.

We have all heard of baby fat. This is not cellulite but actually, in part, a special kind of fat known as brown fat. The pseudo-cellulitic appearance of a baby's arms and legs is mainly due to the high concentration of hyaluronic acid in an infant's skin. A baby's dimple fat gradually disappears after the first six to eight months, as hyaluronic acid decreases. If a baby is improperly fed, however, more fat cells may form and hyaluronic acid may stimulate existing fat cells to enlarge.

Luckily by our teens our "baby fat" is gone. At school and socializing with their friends, teens have a less than optimal diet. Their interpretation of the four major food groups are Wendy's, McDonald's, Burger King, and Pizza Hut! They dine on junk foods filled with sugar, fats, salt and preservatives. Few get sufficient exercise.

Struggling through this stressful stage of life, the teenager, although painfully aware of the physiological changes occurring within her body, does not really understand them. The changes in a girl's body as she grows taller than the boys, develops breasts, and starts her period can and do cause anxiety.

But before too long, menstrual cycles become regular, the girl becomes accustomed to her breasts, and water retention decreases as anovulatory cycles give way to ovulation, permitting progesterone to counteract the estrogen effect. The weight gain caused by estrogen finally hits a plateau. And although it seems as if it will never happen, puberty ends, and a lovely, more confident woman blooms. If at all possible, it is important to intervene quickly at the critical time of puberty to prevent the cycle of cellulite from beginning and increasing. Developing good habits of nutrition and exercise in the teenage years pays dividends for an entire lifetime!

THE PILL

The contraceptive pill, the most widely accepted form of birth-control for women today, is a mixture of two hormones, estrogen and progesterone. The ratio of these very hormones, you will recall, affects fat storage and water retention. Over the last decade, the composition of the Pill has been improved, decreasing its estrogen content. For those women who suffer from monthly menstrual cramps, the Pill can provide welcome relief. But for all of its benefits, the Pill can also have disturbing side effects.

The most common complaints are weight gain, water retention, and a contribution to the development of cellulite. Another side effect, which often occurs years later, is the development of spider veins on the legs. Some women can also have anovulatory cycles for several years after they discontinue the Pill, making it difficult to conceive.

PREGNANCY

I have a bit of good news: during pregnancy, particular hormones actually retard the formation of cellulite, which means that all the water and weight gain may not have a permanent effect. But this does not mean that you shouldn't be careful. Subject always to following your doctor's advice closely, the best precautions to take during this time are to avoid very salty foods, control excessive weight gain, keep your feet elevated and wear support stockings, especially during the last trimester.

MATURITY

Sophie Tucker once said, "From birth to 18 a girl needs good parents. From 18 to 35 she needs good looks. From 35 to 55 she needs a good personality, and from 55 on she needs cash." That may have been the belief in the 1940s, but it's not true

today. Women in their fifties and beyond are having fuller, more productive and enjoyable lives than ever before. We always need our good looks, (though having some cash doesn't hurt!)

Many people believe that ageing is merely a state of mind. In some cases this is true, but try to explain that to your thighs! A word of caution: as we approach and pass 50, cellulite can creep up on us, slowly and quietly. This is because as we grow older, the body's metabolism slows down unless we make regular exercise a part of our daily routine.

This book is written for women of all ages. Lucille Ball offered anti-ageing advice to a friend of mine. She said, "The secret to staying young is to eat slowly, live honestly, and lie about your age." By integrating my simple plan into your daily life, regardless of your age you will discover a fountain of youth that will renew your body, spirit and figure.

MENOPAUSE

Many women are depressed by the prospect of the menopause; the dreaded "change" is approached with anxiety and trepidation. However, the thought that menopause means you are no longer attractive is a lot of bunk. I offer the examples of our not-over-the-hill sisters Jane Fonda, Joan Collins, Linda Evans, and Raquel Welch! Now don't think, "They're wealthy. They have the time, and they can afford to work out daily." My reply is, "Can you afford not to?" Believe me, if you follow the program in this book, you can look and feel every bit as good!

Menopause is actually a time of life when you should have the time of your life. You've raised your children and/or survived career changes, and now the prospect of a bit more leisure or discretionary time should excite you. You now have the luxury of being able to care about yourself. Many women mistakenly feel menopause might rob them of their womanly wiles, that their lives are half over; yet menopause should be thought of as a time of great freedom and reward. Your sexual attraction remains intact and the enjoyment is present without the panic of possible pregnancy. One actress says it's a time "when that little white pill you take just before sex is usually an aspirin."

But what happens in our battle against cellulite during menopause? Here's the good news! Without the high levels of estrogen and the frequent anovulatory cycles preceding menopause causing the imbalance of female hormones, there is less water retention and less formation of cellulite. But please, do not be misled by this small gift. It is still important to continue to exercise daily, not only to prevent the loss of muscle, but also to help in the prevention of osteoporosis (excessive loss of bone mass). Supplemental hormone treatments and calcium tablets can often be useful in deterring this condition. Do check with your physician.

ETHNIC AND GENETIC VARIABLES

As chronicled in Chapter 1, artists have depicted cellulite on the thighs, hips, stomachs and buttocks of the most beautiful women. Venus was the Goddess of Love, not the Fountain of Flab, yet look at the cellulite on her tummy!

Scientific studies of both men and women the world over – in China, Egypt, Brazil, Mexico, Afghanistan, Russia, Japan, Thailand, Indonesia, Italy and Spain, for example – demonstrate that cellulite is observed in all cultures and races. Drs. Nuremberger and Muller studied the Bantus in South Africa and discovered that even their statuesque women have cellulite.

Genetics and racial characteristics, however, do play a part in the amount and location of cellulite on the female body. For example, cellulite is more frequently found among Mediterranean women than in the Nordic or the Oriental populations. The reason may be found in their respective diets! The Nordic people eat large quantities of fish and fruits, while southerly cultures dine on more animal fats, as in lamb and beef. Certain peoples – Jews and Italians, for example – are more likely to treat the meal as a primary social ritual, bringing the family together. (I dare you to have dinner in a Jewish household and try to eat "just a little." And after one full meal of traditional Italian cuisine, it takes an average of two days to feel hungry again!) As the Japanese have gradually changed to a more Western diet, their incidence not only of heart attack but also of cellulite has increased.

Genetics and individual family-inherited traits play an important role as well in both the amount of cellulite you may develop and where it is located on your body. Chances are, if your mother had cellulite, you are a prime candidate and should guard against it.

BODY WEIGHT

"I'm happy with my weight. It keeps me warm, it keeps me company and it keeps my pants up." "I'm not overweight, I'm big-boned." "Fat people are jolly." "I'm built for comfort, not for speed."

These are all cute phrases, but they are rarely uttered with sincerity. Surveys indicate that over 90 percent of women in the United States are not happy with the appearance of their bodies. However, sometimes we apologize to ourselves for the condition of our bodies only to put off our starting to improve them. Remember that being overweight or obese not only has potentially severe psychological ramifications, but may also cause many serious health problems.

Chapter 2 explains that women have fat cells packaged within sacs of connective tissue. Any increase in weight increases the size of each fat cell. With extreme weight gain, even more fat cells can form. No

matter how or why the weight is gained, the dimpling effect of cellulite inevitably results. As we have learned, with time the pressure of the enlarged fat cells in the confined space of their connective tissue sacs causes a change in the capillaries, in turn decreasing the flow of blood and exacerbating the cellulite.

All women who are overweight have obvious, lumpy cellulite. Woman at their optimal weight or thinner have less visible cellulite on their thighs, buttocks or abdomen, though it can clearly be a problem in a non-toned body. Controlling your weight is therefore critical. You will learn easy, effective ways to do so in my *Simple Steps to Thin Thighs* program.

DIET

If you have bounced from diet to diet in attempts to lose weight, you will know there is no better way to break the "pound barrier" than through healthful nutrition. So why are you overweight?

Perhaps you eat too much; or maybe you don't eat too much but you eat poorly. (A good rule is never eat more than you can lift!) You may consume too many fats or too much sugar. It's possible that you don't eat balanced meals, or that you snack or graze all day long. Preparing meals for your family or packing a lunch for yourself may tempt you to taste everything and not waste those leftovers. (My friend's mother prepared *all* her family meals from leftovers. Apparently the original meal has never been found!) Come to think of it, what are you feeding your children? It's important to give children nutritious diets consisting of few refined sugars and minimal fats because during their growth cycles each fat cell increases with weight gain, and weight gain in turn promotes more and more fat cells. Once established, this pattern for weight gain can often recur later in life.

Are you a "salt-oholic"? All adults should avoid extra salt! Not only does salt cause water to accumulate temporarily between the fat cells, slowing the flow of blood and causing changes in the capillary structure, but it also stimulates you to eat more – contributing to long-term weight gain. Even if you don't salt your food, be aware of hidden salts in the foods you eat. Cheese is a particular villain, as are canned soups, canned vegetables, soft drinks, diet sodas, and luncheon meats. Particular care should be taken when ordering at restaurants. All these facts are discussed in detail in Chapter 7, and not all the diet tips in Chapter 7 are about what to avoid. You will also learn how to eat to actually help fat move out of fat cells!

EXERCISE

There's no doubt that you can change your body's shape through exercise. Whether moderate exercise does actually increase the metabolic rate or just promote fat loss is at present a controversial subject. Some forms of exercise may increase total body weight by increasing muscle mass and replacing fat tissue. Generally this is good, but some exercises that increase muscle can also make cellulite more noticeable by pushing the muscle against the fat packages below the skin's surface. The best way to decrease the appearance of cellulite is to *stretch* the muscles – to elongate the body. In Chapter 8 you will learn a fabulous routine of the very best exercises that will make your body slimmer in appearance in just weeks. And this routine takes only minutes a day!

BLOOD CIRCULATION

When we think of our weight problems, we often ignore our circulatory system. Rarely do we stop to think of how our blood is pumping through our veins and feeding all our body's cells, much less of our circulation having anything to do with our fat. We tend to think of fat as the result of a binge on pizza, potato chips, or chocolate chip ice cream, never stopping anywhere in our bodies but making a direct bee-line to our thighs, bellies and behinds. In fact, our blood carries this fat to these "hot spot" areas.

Although it is not caused by poor blood circulation, cellulite, once in place for a period of time, can slow down your circulation. And any long-term condition that compromises the flow of blood within your body can in turn aggravate existing cellulite, making it appear worse. Your circulation can also be restricted by girdles, tight belts, skin-tight jeans and bras that are too small. Although it is unlikely that overly tight clothing can cause serious long-term hindrance to blood circulation, it most assuredly does not help the blood flow to the subcutaneous tissue where your cellulite lives.

Another culprit that adversely affects your blood flow is poor posture. Wearing high heels or uncomfortable shoes can alter your stance. The added weight of pregnancy can make you stoop. Working at a desk with poor lighting or leaning towards a computer screen can cause you to slump. Regularly checking and correcting your body-alignment not only elongates your body, making cellulite less noticeable, but also helps to decrease the possibility of compromised blood flow to the areas where cellulite could accumulate. Methods to help your health and appearance by improving your posture are described in Chapter 8. Mother was right when she constantly nagged you to "stand up straight"! Good posture alone can make you appear slimmer instantly!

PSYCHOLOGICAL CONSIDERATIONS

It is not uncommon for women to surrender to or even begrudgingly make friends with their fat. No one ever said it was easy to lose that excess weight, especially the pudding on your stomach, hips, buttocks and thighs. If you have fought or currently are fighting the "battle

of the bulge," you will know that there are no quick solutions – after all, think how long it took you to gain the weight. It is very important for you to determine *why* you are not slim.

Psychiatrists and psychologists have expounded numerous theories to interpret the "deeper meaning" of women's cellulite. Harboring sexual guilt or not wanting to be close to a partner may induce more cellulite. Perhaps cellulite is a physical cushion to protect women from a hostile or stressful external world, or an out-of-control attempt to develop a more curvaceous, feminine body. Other theories include memories of early childhood emotional pain, holding onto the lumps and bumps of the past, difficulty in moving forward, or fear of choosing a present or future direction. Each of these interpretations as well as many others may or may not apply to any individual.

Perhaps your own honest introspection and meditation will help you discover underlying psychological reasons that contribute to your cellulite. The questionnaires in Chapter 4 may help you find a key which unlocks the door to losing your unwanted cellulite more rapidly. And the information in Chapter 6 will give you the tools to restructure any negative, self-defeating thoughts into positive concepts that stay with you, to make action easy. The point is, whatever your type of frame and whatever your frame of mind, you can do it!

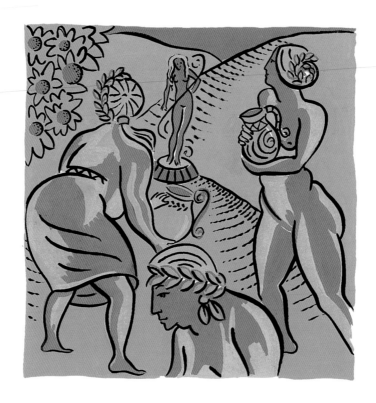

Personal
body analysis

O n the following pages are three extensive questionnaires
regarding your weight, your diet, and your exercise routine. Take
time to answer these questions honestly. Thinking about your
responses and committing them to writing offers you valuable self-
analysis – better than a session with a psychologist or psychiatrist.
Through these questionnaires you will know yourself better; you will

recognize your motivations; you will discover the patterns of your habits; you will understand how your family, friends and role models have influenced you both in the past and present. You will uncover emotions that influence your food cravings and your feelings about exercise.

Take this time to understand the link between your motivations and ingrained habits and your actions. You will find yourself more in control. The rest of this book will provide a method which you will personalize, tailoring a routine and healthy eating habits to suit you individually.

YOUR REFLECTION REACTION

How do you really feel about your body? Now is the time for you to evaluate yourself honestly in the privacy of your home, being sure not to be *too* critical. Remember, attractive bodies come in all sizes and shapes. If you can establish your own ideal, you can be sure that your efforts will not go unnoticed or unappreciated.

For the Weight History questionnaire, you will weigh yourself and list the areas on your body which have cellulite. Then you will actually begin your improvement by doing the most important test of all: The Reflection Reaction. Look at yourself in the mirror to judge whether the dimply appearance of cellulite is terrible (+3), bad (+2), minimal (+1), or non-existent. Your goal should be simply to demonstrate to yourself that you improve. You will be proud of your ever-better reflection.

THE QUESTIONNAIRES

Your first step is to measure your waist, hips and thighs, as indicated below in the illustration and to record the results on the chart overleaf.

Measure your waist; hips (at the widest point); right and left upper thighs (at the top of the inner thigh); right and left mid thighs 6 inches (15 cm) below the upper thigh measurement; and right and left low thighs (just above the knee bone). Repeat these measurements every four weeks. Although each measurement may change only a little and some not at all, each month you will be happy to see a loss in the sum of all measurements. Your goal will be to lose about 1-2 inches (2.5-5 cm) in the sum of your measurements.

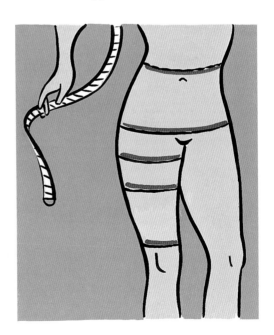

DATE _____	WAIST _____	UPPER THIGH • RIGHT _____	LEFT _____
WEIGHT _____	HIP _____	MID THIGH • RIGHT	LEFT _____
OVERALL REFLECTION REACTION _____	(inches or cm)	LOW THIGH • RIGHT	LEFT _____

Record your measurements here and in the Weekly Review Chart on page 124.

WEIGHT HISTORY

1. Age _____   Height _____   Present weight _____   Desired weight _____

2. Which areas of your body have cellulite? List your Reflection Reaction — whether you consider your cellulite in each area to be terrible (+3), bad (+2), minimal (+1), or none?

arms____   back____   stomach____   outer thigh____   inner thigh____   knee____   buttocks____

However bad you consider your cellulite to be, you will improve by following the Simple Steps to Thin Thighs plan described in this book.

3. How would you describe your present weight?

| | UNDERWEIGHT | | | OVERWEIGHT | |
| **Very** | **Slightly** | **Just Right** | **Slightly** | **Very** |

How do your family/friends describe your weight?

| | UNDERWEIGHT | | | OVERWEIGHT | |
| **Very** | **Slightly** | **Just Right** | **Slightly** | **Very** |

As long as the weight you desire is within 10 percent of the normal weight for your height and build, don't let the opinions of others put pressure on you. Just be comfortable with yourself.

4. How much does your weight fluctuate?

each day?_____   each week? _____   each month? _____

Would a weight fluctuation of 5 lb (2.3 kg) affect the way you feel about yourself?_____
Do you think too much **about food?** _____   **about dieting?** _____

Everyone's weight fluctuates in the course of each day, each week, and each month. Try not to become obsessed with these variances. If you are preoccupied with dieting, if you find that your mood is defined by your precise weight at any given moment, my advice is "relax; go easy on yourself; don't become a victim of your weight." Just concentrate on enjoying food and exercise, and your weight loss will follow naturally.

5. List your maximum weight for each age and how many pounds (or kg) you may have considered yourself to be overweight.

Age	Max. Weight	Llbs Over	Age	Max. Weight	Llbs Over
15-20	_____	_____	40-45	_____	_____
20-25	_____	_____	45-50	_____	_____
25-30	_____	_____	50-55	_____	_____
30-35	_____	_____	55-60	_____	_____
35-40	_____	_____	60-65	_____	_____

Be lenient with yourself in considering how much overweight you were or are. Do check with the desirable weight chart shown on page 47 and aim for a weight at which you will be comfortable and happy and healthy.

6. When did you first start putting on excess weight?

	Yes	No
Infancy	____	____
Childhood (5-12 years old)	____	____
Puberty	____	____
When you moved home	____	____
Marriage	____	____
With the birth of your children	____	____
Menopause	____	____
After a hysterectomy or other surgery	____	____
With emotional stress (1) Family illness	____	____
(2) Death of family or friend	____	____
(3) Divorce or separation	____	____
(4) Difficulty with job	____	____
(5) Other emotional strain	____	____
With diagnosis of a disease: thyroid disease, diabetes, hormonal imbalance revealed by blood tests	____	____

Perhaps now you will realize that some specific event in your life triggered a weight change.

7. Does anyone in your family have a history of being overweight or having cellulite?

	Approx. lb (kg) overweight	Areas with cellulite
Mother	_____	_____
Sister(s)	_____	_____
Children	_____	_____
Brother(s)	_____	
Father	_____	

In any family tending to overweight or to cellulite the cause is partly genetic and partly due to eating and exercise habits. Even if your genetics seem against you, new habits can help.

8.. Do you want to lose weight?   **Yes | No** List your three most important reasons.

1. _____
2. _____
3. _____

It is always easy to list the first reason: you want to look better, perhaps for a specific occasion or for a special person, or you want to be healthier. The other two reasons may be more difficult to name: they may represent more subconsciously profound reasons. As you improve, keep all these reasons in your mind as special goals.

9. Do your family and friends express opinions about your losing weight?

Disapprove _____ **No opinion** _____ **Encouraging** _____

Beware of those who try to "help" by discouraging you and accept with joy all the encouragement you can get!

10. Do you have any medical problems that are complicated by your weight?

	Yes	No
Arthritis	____	____
Foot, knee, leg, back injury	____	____
Bruising	____	____
Diabetes	____	____
Hypertension	____	____
Thrombophlebitis	____	____
Heart disease	____	____
Hyperlipidemia	____	____
Sleep disturbance	____	____

If you have any of these problems, it really will help to attain an acceptable weight.

DIET HISTORY

1. Do you regularly eat?

	AMOUNT OF					AMOUNT OF		
	Yes/No	Small	Medium	Large		Yes/No	Small	Medium	Large
Breakfast	___	___	___	___	Morning snack	___	___	___	___
Lunch	___	___	___	___	Afternoon snack	___	___	___	___
Cocktails	___	___	___	___	Dinner	___	___	___	___
Evening snack	___	___	___	___	Late night snack	___	___	___	___

More meals are better - as long as they are not huge and full of fatty foods. Beware of the extra calories in alcohol and the snacks that often accompany it.

2. Do you regularly have dessert?

	Yes/No	Type	Amount/day
	___	___	___

Learn to choose fruit, not fatty, sugary desserts.

3. Do you drink alcohol with meals? | ___ | ___ | ___ |

between meals? | ___ | ___ | ___ |

You do not need all those extra calories!

4. Do you drink caffeinated drinks (coffee, tea)? | ___ | ___ | ___ |

Caffeine itself is not bad (unless you react badly to it, e.g. palpitations). Just don't drink too much!

5. Do you smoke? | ___ | ___ | ___ |

Smoking is really unhealthy! It makes your skin prematurely age, giving wrinkles and extra, unattractive blood vessels - and it causes lung cancer. If you smoke, you should use this improvement time to quit and change to healthy habits!

6. Do you have the same eating habits as your parents?   **Yes | No**
Is what you eat influenced by:
your family? ___   **your roommate?** ___   **your friends?** ___

Make this the time to choose your own good habits; do not simply follow the bad habits of people around you.

7. Do you binge **Yes | No** when you are: **nervous and under pressure?** _____
happy? _____ **sad?** _____ **angry?** _____ **alone?** _____ **bored?** _____
procrastinating with other tasks? _____ **on weekends?** _____ **on holidays?** _____
at Christmas / Easter / other celebrations? _____

Perhaps your eating relates not to your hunger but to your emotions.

8. Do you eat just before you go to bed?   **Yes | No**
Do you have trouble falling asleep at night? _____ **getting up in the morning?** _____
Do you have trouble sleeping through the night? _____

Perhaps you will realize that your midnight snack either upsets or helps your sleep.

9. How often have you thought about losing weight?

Never	Every few months	Every year	Every few years	All the time

How often have you gone on a diet to lose weight?

Never	Every few months	Every year	Every few years	All the time

The eating plan you will learn here will free you from diets and from worry about your weight.

10. What have you done to lose weight?
Was it successful long-term?

	When	Precise method	Successful Yes	No
Do-it-yourself diet	_____	_____	___	___
Supervised diet (doctor, nutritionist, program)	_____	_____	___	___
Very-low-calorie diet**	_____	_____	___	___
Fasting**	_____	_____	___	___
Behavior modification	_____	_____	___	___
Hypnosis	_____	_____	___	___
Psychiatric or psychological consultation	_____	_____	___	___
Diet pills*	_____	_____	___	___
Diuretics*	_____	_____	___	___
Laxatives*	_____	_____	___	___
Self prescribed medications*	_____	_____	___	___
Self-induced vomiting*	_____	_____	___	___
Exercise program	_____	_____	___	___

*Methods marked with * are unhealthy and should not be used! ** can be risky and not recommended. Combine any methods which worked for you with those described in this book.*

11. Do you take any medications?

Anticoagulants _____   **Blood pressure medication** _____
Diabetes medicine (oral or insulin) _____   **Digitalis** _____
Diuretic _____   **Epilepsy medication** _____
Headache medications _____   **Sleep medications** _____
Heart medications (digoxin, nitroglycerin etc) _____

If you take any of these medicines or others, you must be seen regularly by your physician.

12. Do you have any allergies to any medicines, drugs or foods?   **Yes | No**

Obviously you must avoid any medication or food to which you are allergic!

13. Do you have any diseases which are directly affected by your diet?   **Yes | No**

Allergies ____   **Diabetes** ____   **Headaches** ____   **Heart disease** ____   **Hypertension** ____
Kidney disease ____   **Liver or gall bladder disease** ____   **Mood swings** ____
Sleeping disorder ____   **Ulcers, gastrointestinal disease** ____
Urinary or bladder infection ____

You should consult your physician before beginning any diet or exercise program. If you have any of the above conditions, be sure to discuss your plan with your doctor before starting.

EXERCISE HISTORY

1. I don't exercise because:

I just don't have time! ____
I am too heavy and awkward to be seen exercising! ____
I have exercised before, and I did not lose one pound! ____
I get all the exercise I need keeping up with my children! ____
I can't exercise - it makes me sweaty and tired! ____
I could hurt myself jogging! ____
It's too cold (hot) to start exercising now! I'll wait until summer (winter)! ____

There is no good excuse not to start now!

2. How active are you?   **Very inactive   Inactive   Average   Active   Very active**

You don't need to exercise for hours each day. Thirty minutes, five times a week is an optimal amount of exercise for the average person.

3. What do you do for physical exercise and how often do you do it?
If you could do anything, what exercise would you do and how often would you do it?

	ACTIVITY	FREQUENCY			ACTIVITY	FREQUENCY
Do:				**Desire:**		

Keep doing what you are doing and take the time to add the exercise you really want to do even if that requires a training period or equipment. Your health is worth it!

4. Did family/friends/role models exercise regularly as you were growing up?
Do they now? If so, identify the person/people and the exercise.

When growing up   **Now**

You may be surprised to see how the people around you have influenced you. Learn from everyone! Adopt the good habits of your role models and discard the defeatist habits of others.

5. Did you ever exercise regularly or play sports?

Age	Exercise	Age	Exercise
5-15		30-40	
15-20		40-50	
20-25		50-60	
25-30		Over 60	

You are never too old to start exercising! Any increase in exercise helps. Remember "Don't lie down when you can sit; don't sit when you can stand; don't stand when you can walk/move."

6. Do you want to exercise more?   **Yes | No**   List your three most important reasons.

1. _____
2. _____
3. _____

Everyone can find 12 minutes each day! You can exercise in your own home!

7. How many hours do you watch television **each day?** _____ **each week?** _____

Don't be a couch potato! You can always exercise in front of the TV!

8. Do your family and friends express opinions about your exercising?

      Disapprove _____ **No opinion** _____ **Encouraging** _____

It's easier to exercise with a friend. If anyone discourages you, remember it is your time.

9. Do you have any disease that hinders your exercise? **Yes | No**

Adrenal disorder _____ **Anemia** _____ **Arthritis** _____
Blood or clotting disorders; bruising _____ **Convulsions** _____
Diabetes _____ **Foot, knee, back injury** _____ **Heart disease** _____
Hormonal disorder _____ **Hyperlipidemia** _____ **Hypertension** _____
Asthma _____ **Lung disease; bronchitis** _____ **Tuberculosis** _____
Thrombophlebitis _____ **Thyroid disorder** _____

Ask your doctor about the type and amount of exercise recommended for you.

10. Did anyone in your family have a heart attack or stroke before they were 50 years old? If so, at what age?

Mother _____ **Father** _____ **Sister** _____ **Brother** _____ **Grandparent** _____

If you are over 40 years old or if anyone in your family had a heart attack, do check with your physician before starting any exercise regime.

11. Do you have any of these symptoms? **Yes | No**

Abdominal pain _____ **Back pain, ankle pain, shoulder or arm pain** _____
Breathlessness with exertion _____ **Chest pain** _____ **Coughing** _____
Coughing blood _____ **Dizziness** _____ **Fainting** _____
Hot flashes _____ **Inappropriate coldness** _____
Inappropriate drowsiness _____ **Palpitations** _____ **Swollen joint** _____

If you have any of these symptoms or anything else which worries you, then consult your doctor before beginning any new diet or exercise program.

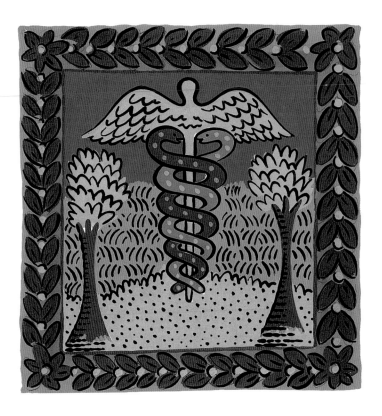

What your doctor can do

E very one of us should have a physician whom we know and trust. The secret to good health is knowing when and how to consult that physician for medical advice. Even when you think you are completely healthy, it is advisable to have an annual physical examination. After all, you take your car for an inspection even when there is nothing wrong. Don't you owe yourself an equal courtesy for your very own body? Your most important duty in life is to attain your highest potential, which you can only achieve by maintaining your good health.

How an Examination Helps

We are the healthiest people in all of history; we have the best diagnostic tools and the most sophisticated treatments ever. Unfortunately most of us use these advantages not for "health care," but only "disease care" – we go to a physician just to fix our ailments. In certain societies in Asia, the village doctor's task is simply to keep people healthy. She or he is paid only when the patients are well; when they are sick, this "wellness doctor" must restore health before being compensated. So use your physician as a "wellness doctor"!

You should keep track each year of some of the measurements your doctor makes – such as your regular resting pulse rate, your blood pressure, your weight, your levels of blood glucose, triglyceride, and total cholesterol as well as HDL and LDL cholesterol.

Your physician can also check other factors that can affect your energy, your weight, and your metabolism. Routine blood tests can check for anemia, thyroid disorder, and whether your liver and kidneys are functioning properly.

Other than your annual physical, the other time to check with your doctor when you are healthy is when you embark on a significant change in your lifestyle, such as

when you begin a diet and/or exercise program. Be sure that your physician approves of this regime for you. The guidance in this book is not meant as a substitute for your physician's advice.

Obviously, if you have *any symptoms* such as those listed in the diet and exercise questionnaires in Chapter 4, you must seek medical advice. You are not alone; your doctor can help!

Do You Have Unhealthy Fat?

The conventional way to determine optimal weight has been with tables showing "standard" weights for differing heights and body frames (determined by wrist size). However, in my opinion the current tables do not reflect the weights to which we should aspire to look and feel our best; the weights are a bit high and are getting higher. In comparing the tables from 1983 with those of 1959 (see page 47), "ideal" weights have increased 2 percent (for tall women) to 10 percent (for short women).

The other major limitation with these tables is that weight does not reflect fatness. A trained athlete and a person of the same height who sits all day in front of the television can be the same weight, but their bodies will most likely look quite different! We must worry not about being overweight, but about being *over fat*. The body is composed of lean mass (muscle, bones, organs) and fat mass. About 36 percent of a woman's weight is muscle and 12 percent is bone. Absolutely essential fat surrounding all cells, nerves, and organs is about three percent of body weight for men and about 12 percent of body weight for women. This higher value for women includes the fat deposited at puberty in the breasts and – sigh – the hips.

The optimal range of body fat for women is 15-25 percent of body weight. Under 12 percent fat is not healthy and may be associated with serious eating disorders such as anorexia nervosa or bulimia – seen increasingly in young women whose distorted body images drive them to self-induced, alarming emaciation. In women, over 30 percent fat is not healthy, and over 35 percent signals definite medical risks.

Women can roughly estimate their percentage of fat, by using the nomogram on page 47. (A similar nomogram for men uses weight and waist girth.) For a more accurate measurement of your percentage of fat your doctor may be able to help. Until recently, this could be done only in special facilities because a person had to be weighed completely submerged in water. Remember Archimedes' Principle? The Greek mathematician Archimedes realized that when he got into a bath, the level of water rose equal to the volume of his submerged body. To calculate percentage of fat, body volume can be measured by seeing how much less the person weighs in water than in air. Using the difference in density of fat and muscle (0.9 versus 1.1 grams per milliliter,

respectively), the percentage of body fat can be calculated. (Because of this slight difference in density, a fat person can float easily and a very muscular person sinks!)

Today your doctor can measure body composition quite easily using a method called bioelectric impedance. With simple sensors on the wrist and on the foot, conductance is measured painlessly, without disrobing and getting all wet! Percentage fat is calculated automatically within seconds, taking into account age, sex, height and weight.

Knowing your body composition gives you great incentive to lose fat and to gain muscle. Not only will you see your firmer, thinner body as you follow the program you are about to learn, but also your doctor can measure your improvement!

LIPOSUCTION

Even if a woman is not overweight and if she does successfully decrease the dimpling appearance of her cellulite by the methods described in this book, she may still be plagued by unsightly deposits of fat, especially on her hips (aptly called "saddlebags") or thighs ("jester's pants"), her lower back ("love handles"), her stomach or above her knees.

Unfortunately, some women are born with extra fat cells in these particular areas, a genetic condition known medically as lipodysmorphia. Although diet, exercise, and massage may decrease these bulges they may stubbornly remain.

Fortunately, liposuction – the technique of surgical removal of these fat deposits – has been perfected in recent years. Unlike the first buttock lift operation by Dr. John R. Lewis in Atlanta, Georgia (1957) and the first surgical removal of fat from thighs by Dr. Ivo Pittanguy in Rio de Janeiro (1958), which left long scars from the excisions, the new technique is done by vacuuming fat from under the skin through a small incision, leaving only a tiny scar. This method was first introduced in France in the mid 1970s by Dr. Yves Gerard Illouz and has been improved by French and American plastic surgeons. Now more than 100,000 American women have body liposuction each year. In fact, this operation is becoming the most popular surgical procedure in America.

Liposuction is a relatively simple procedure. With the patient under either general anesthesia or heavy sedation, the surgeon makes a small incision (about ¼ inch/6 mm) within the natural crease of the skin in the site to be trimmed. Then a cannula – a metal tube with several holes on one side – is inserted and attached to a vacuum pump. The surgeon moves the cannula back and forth, literally sucking out the fat. The procedure takes less than one hour. The patient usually goes home that day with the area tightly bandaged to prevent the accumulation of fluid. Healing takes four to six weeks, during which the patient is advised to wear a support girdle. Although she must rest for a few days and

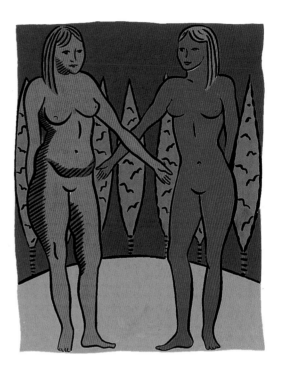

The areas most commonly treated by liposuction are the inner and outer thighs, the buttocks, the stomach, the lower back, occasionally the knees (shown by shaded areas), and rarely the upper arms.

there is severe bruising, she can resume her normal activities in several days and her usual exercise routine within one week.

With liposuction, the body is literally sculpted so that unattractive fat deposits are gone! Most patients are thrilled because their jeans size decreases and their body silhouette has contour instead of bulges. However, a liposuction patient can and will gain weight if she begins to overeat and does not exercise. The difference in weight gain is that instead of having extra-large deposits of fat in the areas suctioned, her added weight will first be distributed proportionately over all of her remaining fat cells. Until recently it was thought that once fat cells have been removed, they would not grow back. Now we know this is not true. There are tiny, unfilled fat cells along the capillaries (small blood vessels) just waiting for fat to be delivered from the blood. When fat is eaten, these gobble up that fat to form new fat cells. So to keep the improved contour, it is absolutely necessary to eat a low-fat diet and to exercise.

Liposuction cannot be used as a quick fix for obesity. Only about one to three pounds (0.4-1.4 kg) of fat are actually removed with this procedure. In fact, any patient who is overweight is sent home to diet and exercise before she can be considered for surgical suctioning. The ideal candidate for liposuction is within 10 percent of her ideal weight with only localized fat deposits. Women (and men) of any age can have liposuction as long as they are in good health and have good skin tone, since the skin must be elastic enough to contract over the suctioned area. Because the skin on the arm is especially prone to sagging after liposuction, this is rarely done to the arms.

There are, however, a few adverse side effects after liposuction. Although small and camouflaged in the skin folds, there are scars. There is always swelling and soreness just after the surgery which

resolves within days, and bruising which resolves within one month. Any long-term darkening of the skin can be medically treated. Occasionally the skin sags, or there are uneven ripples of the surface. This can easily be corrected surgically. There is a slight risk of numbing of the skin over the suctioned site, a condition that is usually temporary but (in rare cases) can last years.

This surgery should be considered as a last resort, only after you have faithfully followed the *Simple Steps to Thin Thighs* program for several months and remain dissatisfied. Be sure of your motivation; liposuction should not be done frivolously. Surgery does not reshape your life – it simply resculpts your body contours, and only successfully if you are not very overweight. It is vital to choose an experienced surgeon who clearly evaluates you personally and does not promise a miracle.

For many, liposuction eliminates the long-despised bulges of fat but it is no substitute for a healthy diet and exercise plan. Follow the *Simple Steps to Thin Thighs* program described in Chapters 7, 8 and 9 and then decide!

Top right: from Desirable Weights for Women from "New Weight Standards for Men and Women" by the Metropolitan Life Insurance Company of New York, 1959 Statistical Bulletin, 40 pp1-4.

Bottom right: Fat Percentage Nomogram: adapted from Wilmore, J.H., (1986). "Sensible Fitness"; Champaign, Ill.: Human Kinetics.

■ Desirable Weights for Women (25 years and over)

Height (ft/ins)	Weight in pounds		
	small frame	medium frame	large frame
4'8"	92-98	96-107	104-119
4'9"	94-101	98-110	106-122
4'10"	96-104	101-113	109-125
4'11"	99-107	104-116	112-128
5'0"	102-110	107-119	115-131
5'1"	105-113	110-122	118-134
5'2"	108-116	113-126	121-138
5'3"	111-119	116-130	125-142
5'4"	114-123	120-135	129-146
5'5"	118-127	124-139	133-150
5'6"	122-131	128-143	137-154
5'7"	126-135	132-147	141-158
5'8"	130-140	136-151	145-163
5'9"	134-144	140-155	149-168
5'10"	138-148	144-159	153-173
5'11"	142-152	148-163	157-178
6'0"	146-156	152-167	161-183

Height without shoes. For women aged 18-25 subtract 1lb for every year below 25.
To convert to stone divide by 14.
To convert to kg divide by 2.205.

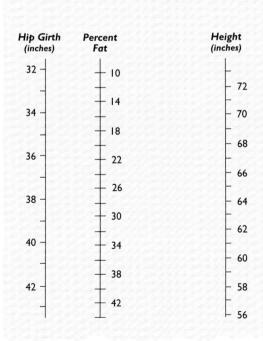

■ Fat Percentage Nomogram

Measure your height (without shoes) and your hip girth at the widest point. On the nomogram draw a straight line between the measurements. Your approximate percent body fat is where the line crosses the middle scale.

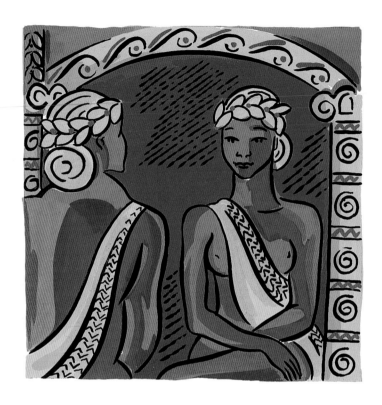

The battle for your brain

D o you really and truly want to lose your cellulite? It's all in the Battle for your Brain! Against you are the Forces of Fat, not very impressive opponents, armed only with the ignorance upon which bad habits are inadvertently formed. By reading this book, you've acquired an invincible tactical plan. "If there is a Why, there is always a How," said Nietzsche. You've determined the "Why" in Chapter 4's

Personal Body Analysis, by listing the reasons for reducing your cellulite, reasons which must be your own, not because your friends, family or doctor insist that you diet or exercise. As to the "How", your ultimate weapon in winning this battle is knowledge: recognizing your enemy, your goals, and what motivates you, and learning the right action to achieve your objectives. Here are a few tips to help you along the road to success. It will be fun, and much easier than you ever imagined!

YOUR TURNING POINT

Your Turning Point is *now*! Think of some event that really made you want to lose your cellulite - a point at which you said, "This is the last straw!" These were the turning points for some of my friends:

"I always wore size 12 slacks, but a saleswoman offered me size 14 – and even they were snug!"

"My colleague stared with amazement at the size of my second helping."

"My eight-year old son and his giggling friend have named my thighs 'Squiggly.'"

Your Turning Point galvanizes vague motivation into lasting commitment. With commitment like this, you can't be beat!

SETTING YOUR GOALS

In Chapter 4 you set down answers that gave you a new, clearer understanding of your attitudes towards yourself. Now you must set your goals – your own realistic, measurable and attainable goals. "Nothing

happens unless first a dream," said the poet Carl Sandburg. When it comes to your body, what are your dreams? That you will fit into those slacks that were perfect a few years ago? That your thighs will look great in your new bathing suit?

Be specific! Committing your goals to writing in your Cellulite Reduction Diary (Chapter 10) makes you really think about them. It's a contract with yourself. Consider in some detail what you want most to improve - the cellulite on your thighs or arms, or those "love handles." Record the weight you want to be.

Be realistic! If your initial goals are beyond the achievable (too much, too soon), you will be discouraged when you fall short and you may even give up. Now that just won't do! For example, if you have a heavier bone structure, don't aim to become petite in build. (Neither should you weigh appreciably less than your "normal" weight - see chart on page 47.)

Be patient! Don't expect your body to be transformed after only a few days. Remember, it took you years to acquire the figure you now have; it will be at least two to four weeks before the improvement in that stubborn cellulite is really apparent. If you are 30 or 40 pounds (14 or 18 kg) overweight, you must lose that weight slowly and steadily over several months. A good goal is to lose about 2 pounds (1 kg) each week; don't be discouraged by a plateau or even a 1 or 2 pound (0.5 or 1 kg) increase on any given day. (Such a fluctuation is really quite natural.)

Build slowly! If you have not been exercising regularly, you cannot expect to launch right into an aerobic program of 20 or 30 minutes, or accomplish all your exercises perfectly on the first go or without pausing. Set small, incremental goals for each day and for each week. Write these down in your diary! Each day, do a little more than the day before.

Set deadlines! Once you've established realistic goals, set for yourself realistic deadlines – not vague ones, but "today," "this week," "this month." Make the pledge that you'll look good in your new, short skirt at your class reunion next month or at the office party. The deadlines will "keep you honest" and on track.

Keep it up! Once you've achieved those important short-term goals, make sure you set new ones so that you can keep moving in the right direction. Thereafter, set your goals in terms of monitoring and maintaining, as well as improving. If you slack off, so will your thighs!

YOUR ACTION PLAN

Now take action! Action is not a gift. You can't buy it; there is no "action gene". We are what we do. Every time we act we strengthen our motivations. Don't procrastinate. Don't buy larger clothes. (That lets you off the hook, giving you a false sense of relief.) Only by taking action can you succeed. Today is the "some day" to begin. Your new plan is outlined clearly in the next three chapters. It's based on science, it's easy, it's fun, and it works! The changing patterns in your life will make you happy, not only with the result but also in the doing.

VISUALIZE THE NEW YOU

You have clarified your goals: you want to be healthy and energetic, with no cellulite – the ideal of today's woman! But you will still be yourself, a unique individual. You need not become super-thin or a marathon athlete. The new you is some combination of what you are now and your image of yourself as you want to be. Visualize that image in detail. You don't want to see ripples when you try on clothes in those over-lit department store dressing rooms. You want sexy thighs without the worry of bumpy cellulite.

Now try something different. Pretend you are that svelte silhouette now! Think of yourself as instantly slimmer, as if you banished your cellulite with the blink of an eye. How would you feel and act? You would consciously and unconsciously feel and act differently, adopting new and healthy habits. You would truly enjoy your body and feel good about yourself.

How would you keep that great new figure? You would eat healthy, nourishing, tasty foods, not junky fats. You would enjoy showing off your cellulite-free self by exercising regularly. You would look forward to interests other than eating. At a movie you would concentrate on the film, forgetting the buttered popcorn. At a buffet, you would taste – not overeat – each food. Just follow the saying, "Think Thin Thighs!" If you *really* "think thin," if in your mind you are your stated goal, living that goal in all of your actions, new, positive habits will reflexively become part of your new self and you can "make it come true" in every sense.

THINK SUCCESS

To accomplish anything, you must believe in yourself and in the fact that you can, indeed will, succeed. It is surprising how often we are unable to complete a task that is well within our capabilities just because we haven't prepared ourselves mentally. The Power of Positive Thinking was introduced by Norman Vincent Peale more than 40 years ago. At that time, no one knew of the real-life mechanism underlying his message. Scientists have now shown that our brain chemistry is physically altered by both our positive and negative emotions. Anger or depression, for example, affect specific molecules that act as messengers in our brains, changing how we feel and behave. Nervousness makes our hearts beat rapidly and our hands clammy; real, physical symptoms arising from our emotional state.

Conversely, positive thoughts bring positive emotions. When Norman Cousins contracted a disabling illness against which doctors gave little hope, he did not give up. Learning from other "miraculous"

recoveries, he concluded that positive thinking was the key. He collected every comedy film he could, from Abbott and Costello to the Three Stooges. As he watched them from his hospital bed, laughing despite his pain, his symptoms markedly improved. Not only did he lead a productive life for years thereafter, but he dedicated the rest of his brilliant career to the study of positive thinking, becoming a professor at UCLA's Medical School.

As you implement the plan described over the next few chapters, you too must, in the words of Johnny Mercer's song, "Accentuate the positive!" Believe in your abilities and be aware of your assets – physical, intellectual and spiritual. You have so many fine qualities, some of which you may not always recognize. (Any friend could certainly list them!) Focus on these many good points of your appearance and character. Sophia Loren reportedly believes that "Nothing makes a woman more beautiful than her belief that she is beautiful." That's easy for Sophia Loren to say, but think about it: we have all run across attractive women who are filled with self-doubt and less physically striking women who are full of self-confidence and poise. If you learn to "think beautiful", you'll feel beautiful according to your own definition of "beauty" (which probably includes thin thighs!). In turn, you will radiate that beauty. Armed with a positive attitude, accomplishing your goals – including losing your cellulite – is easy!

51

HABITS – FRIEND OR ENEMY

You don't invite into your home anyone bent on harming you, do you? We all try to surround ourselves with people who care about us. In the same way, you must selectively invite into your home, and into your life, only those habits that are "your friends." That chocolate cake may look tempting, but in fact it is your enemy, as is watching too many sports but playing too few. Examine your habits and *know your friends from your enemies.*

When it comes to selecting habits, be your own boss! Many of your habits are part of your life not because you've consciously adopted them, but because you acquired them from others in your youth. Don't let the rest of your life be influenced by subconscious behavioral patterns. If we are creatures of habit, these habits should be a part of our lives not by coincidence, but by informed decision!

What is a habit? A habit is a pattern of behavior that over time becomes almost involuntary, a customary part of daily routine or a response to a cause such as anxiety or tension. Do you buy a doughnut every morning or nibble on potato chips as you work? Do you drive to the neighborhood shop when you could walk? If you are nervous, is your first reaction to munch on whatever happens to be available? These are the kinds of unwanted habits you can alter if you so desire. Firstly, identify your habits and single out those that are not friendly to your interests. The three questionnaires in Chapter 4 helped you understand some of your underlying motivations. Write them down. If you can identify your patterns of action (or inaction), half the battle is won!

Actively plan a substitute response, an alternative to your involuntary habit. Break the pattern. If you can't resist buying a cake as you pass the bakery, take another route to work. *Never* take second helpings. Don't munch all the time; but set aside periods of the day when you won't eat. If you do snack, keep Happy Hunger Helpers around (see Chapter 7), rather than peanuts or chips. Eat slowly and you will eat less with greater satisfaction. Keep a photo on the refrigerator of yourself when you were slimmer. If you often skip exercise, place your sports gear where you can't miss it, to jog your memory.

Look to the broader picture. As you reach for the dessert (because it's there), think instead how much happier you'll be tomorrow weighing less. Think of the greater long-term pleasure of looking and feeling much better and of the positive consequences of ridding yourself of your cellulite. Whatever habits you labelled "uncontrollable," tastes you termed "addictive," or lapses of energy you called "resting," change these false labels to reflect the new you! You control your tastes; they don't control you. Think of yourself as you are about to be – cellulite free – and self-defeating behavior patterns will no longer be excess baggage.

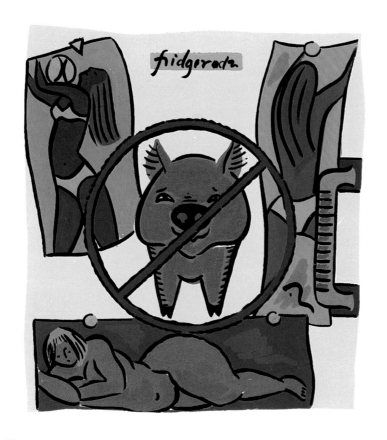

PICTURES HELP!

- *Tape pictures and sayings to your refrigerator to remind you not to overeat.*
- *Keep on your mirror a photo of yourself when you had less cellulite.*
- *Whenever you look at a piece of chocolate cake or an ice cream, visualize a big lump of LARD. That's the fat you're really eating!*
- *Leave on your night table two snapshots – one of your favorite athlete or dancer the other of an overweight person. They will remind you of the effects of exercise on your body!*

REMEMBER!

- *"A moment on your lips, a lifetime on your hips."*
- *"We are all thin people, but some of us are overweight thin people."*
- *"Square meals often make round people." – E. Joseph Cossman*
- *"Every journey, from the shortest to the longest, begins with a first step, followed by another, then another."*
- *"Man begins to achieve when he begins to believe." – J.C. Roberts*

Your personal cellulite reduction program

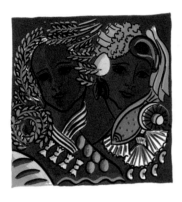

Now that you fully understand the causes and effects of cellulite, here are the solutions!

The following chapters set out the *Simple Steps to Thin Thighs* plan for doing the things to make yourself look and feel better and to make your cellulite disappear. This three-pronged strategy is based on science, it's easy, and you'll enjoy doing it!

First, you will learn to eat to nourish your body – happily, without feeling hunger or unsatisfied cravings. With my GREFLOF, Great Food Low Fat, Plan, you are free to choose the foods you like. You need not follow rigid menus or buy expensive foods in specialty stores. You can eat anywhere – at home with your family or in restaurants – enjoying every meal. You won't become obsessed with a "diet". You need follow only these simple rules:

1. **Avoid fats – especially fat/sugar and fat/salt combinations.**
2. **Feast on certain preferred fruits and vegetables.**
3. **Choose the right kinds of protein in the right combinations.**
4. **You can actually benefit from learning to snack correctly!**
5. **Minimize alcohol to save calories in more ways than one.**
6. **Use artificial sweeteners instead of sugar whenever possible.**
7. **Take the vitamins and minerals that help you lose cellulite.**

"Eat Your Way to a Better You" explains the reasons for these rules and give some fabulous recipes that are easy to prepare and even special enough for guests. The GREFLOF plan will become a way of eating that you will enjoy – and you will be thrilled not only to look better as you shed your unwanted cellulite, but also to feel better – with more energy and vigor, ready for the next part of the program.

Second, you will resculpt your body in only minutes a day – and you will have lots of fun! "A Better Body in Minutes A Day" will lead you step-by-step through a new and different exercise plan. You will learn Pressometrics you can do any time – the Ball Crusher, the Kneecap Kiss, the Flapper – to name just a few. Have you ever been bored in conferences or on telephone calls, impatient as you waited for an elevator or

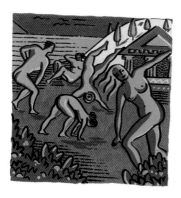

bus, or exasperated when trying to calm your children? Never again! Just smile and secretly do the Suspended Animotion or the Elevator Wait Lift.

With a short routine of Streamline Stretches and the special set of anti-cellulite exercises called the Twelve-Minute Miracle, you will eliminate your unwanted cellulite and at the same time automatically improve your posture, with the result that no matter how you look now, you will look remarkably better very soon. These movements feel so good that they energize you. I look forward to them, and I'm sure you will, too!

Lastly, you will learn to give yourself the luxury of a little time to yourself to move your body in any way you enjoy – walking, swimming, cycling, running, just a few of the many great choices. In front of TV or outside, these aerobics will exhilarate you!

Third, following my advice in Chapter 9, you'll smooth the surface of your skin as you practice the age-old customs of skin brushing and massage. You'll learn about special creams that really can help smooth that uneven, bulging cellulite. These methods will become a part of your life – just like washing your face, and in even less time!

Why do most other diet and exercise plans fail? Because these tough diets are based on denial and deprivation and because rigorous exercise routines take too much time from your already busy schedule. Most programs cannot be followed for very long – barely long enough to start to see improvement, let alone maintain it. When these plans demand too much and fail, you lapse back into your old habits which were themselves responsible for your less-than-perfect health and physique.

If the human race can make it to the moon, we can certainly devise a pain-free system to lose a little cellulite! The strategy you are about to learn feels good, makes you happy and is easy to incorporate into your presently active life. You will chart your progress in your Cellulite Reduction Diary. You will be amazed that you feel so good and look so much better – and have so much fun, with no suffering. You will even wonder how you ever got along before.

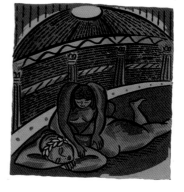

As John Dryden said, "We first make our habits, then our habits make us." With your new knowledge you will easily change your habits so that your body automatically improves. So let's begin!

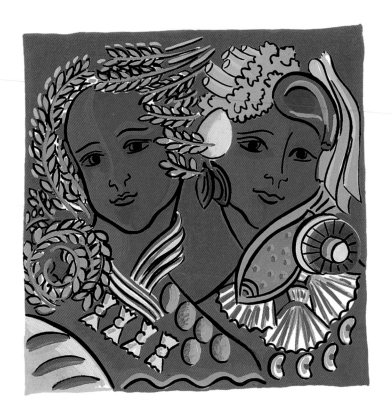

Eat your way
to a better you

When you think about dieting, do you panic? At the prospect of miniscule meals, do you suddenly feel extraordinarily hungry? Do you crave foods you know are fattening? Are you afraid you will not be able to dine out with friends, or eat "normal" meals? With my *Simple Steps to Thin Thighs* eating plan these fears are history! You will learn how food can be true nourishment that will help you in every way. You will enjoy an improved body shape, increased energy and a sense of well-being. And although your primary motivation is most probably to lose your cellulite and look better, you will also become healthier!

Why have your diets failed in the past? Maybe because you felt deprived. You felt hungry or bored; you craved certain foods; you could not follow rigid rules without making great changes to your life-style.

THE GREFLOF EATING PLAN

With my GREFLOF – Great Food, Low Fat – Plan you will learn to attain your ideal weight without deprivation. Believe it or not, this is a never-go-hungry eating plan. And there are other advantages:

1. You don't need foods available only in specialty stores or through specific diet programs. Such food is inconvenient and often expensive; it is also a temporary, artificial way of eating that you cannot reasonably continue throughout your life – especially if you socialize or travel.

2. You needn't count calories or weigh your food – another inconvenience that can make you a mental prisoner of your eating habits. Your mind will be free to enjoy all the other great things in life!

3. You can enjoy delicious meals, eating out or at home. No one will even know that you are eating differently – they will only notice how much better you look!

4. You choose the foods you like to eat. You need not follow rigid menus.

Limit Fats: Fats are Fattening!

Fat adds taste to food along with creamy, hard-to-resist texture. It also slows down digestion so that we feel more satiated; eating a high-fat meal keeps hunger pangs away longer than a low-fat meal.

There is a major downside: with high-fat foods, we eat more calories, even with smaller quantities. Of the three nutrients protein, carbohydrate and fat, fat has the most calories. While one gram of protein or carbohydrate each yield 4 calories, a gram of fat loads you with 9 – and is more easily converted to body fat!

Where is the Fat in our Diet?

We are eating more and more fat because food manufacturers have learned that they can sell more when more fat is added. We eat only about one quarter the amount of butter we did in 1910, but today we eat much more fat in meat and poultry and in processed dairy products such as cheese and ice cream. Animals are purposely fattened before slaughter and extra fat is added to hamburgers and hot dogs. Even supposedly healthy processed foods like granola breakfast bars, yogurt, imitation ice cream and non-dairy coffee whitener are loaded with fat. The real surge, though, has come from "fast foods" in which a healthy, low-fat food like a potato (60 calories and no fat) is transformed into a disastrous helping of French fries (250 calories and 13 grams of fat). Another danger is that many fats are "hidden", like those in processed foods such as cakes, cookies, ice cream and peanut butter.

How much fat should we eat? Experts do not agree! Estimates of the total calories from fat range from 30 per cent (determined by the American Heart Association to reduce atherosclerotic heart disease) to 20 percent to prevent some forms of cancer, to 10 percent or less fat, as recommended by diet gurus, Nathan Pritikin and Dr. Dean Ornish. As a very low fat diet is really quite tough, my recommendation is to aim for a diet of no more than 15 percent fat. What does this mean to you? If you weigh 130 pounds (59 kg), you should eat no more than 32g per day of fat (equal to 290 calories).

However, you do require some fat in your diet. The name of the game is to get your necessary fat from unsaturated sources. There is a simple test that tells you if a fat is saturated or not. If it is solid at room temperature (like the visible fat of meat, butter, lard or cheese) it's saturated; if it is liquid (like vegetable oils) it's unsaturated. With a few exceptions (coconut oil and palm oil), saturated fats are all from animal sources. Beware, though – food processing can actually turn unsaturated vegetable oils into saturated fats. If you use margarines made from vegetable oils, choose the softer ones in the tubs, since they are lower in saturated fats.

The unsaturated fats in your diet should generally be monounsaturated (for example olive and canola oils) which do

not raise blood cholesterol levels, rather than polyunsaturated. A particular group of polyunsaturated fats, however, the fish oils or omega-3 fatty acids found in fish such as salmon, mackerel, herring and trout, help to prevent excessive blood clotting (a factor in heart disease and stroke) when substituted for saturated fatty acids in the diet.

It's easy to cook with very little fat and to use only unsaturated fats. The pages which follow show how to substitute fats without compromising taste!

Fat and Sugar – The Disaster Duo

Do you absolutely adore chocolate or cheesecake? Do you view ice cream as the next thing to heaven? Do you consider yourself a hopeless sugar addict?

Let me reassure you: you do not have an addiction. Nor will you suffer withdrawal from avoiding such foods. You simply have a habit which you need to modify.

What do such foods have in common? They are all made up of about 60 percent sugar and 30 percent fat – 48 percent of their calories are from fat! Why are these foods so disastrous? First and foremost, they taste *delicious*. It's difficult to eat only a little; they slide right down, so we overindulge as a matter of course. Volunteers in scientific studies were asked to make blind taste-tests of various foods and to rate their preferences without knowing what they were eating. Most of these volunteers, whether fat or thin,

EAT YOUR WAY TO A BETTER YOU

preferred a mixture of – guess what – 60 percent sugar and 30 percent fat.

The fact that sugar and fat taste so good is only the start of the disaster! The second and more directly germane problem is that this combination promotes the storage of fat in our bodies. As we eat, the sugar level in our blood rises, thus alerting our pancreas to release insulin to reduce blood-sugar levels. This increased insulin increases our storage of fat! The fat from the sugar-fat mixtures we love to eat, therefore, goes directly to our fat storage depots – our cellulite!

Fat and Salt – Another Disaster

Can you imagine potato chips without salt? Can you ever eat only one salted peanut or corn chip? The problem with these snacks is not the salt, but simply that salt makes high-fat foods taste better so we eat much more.

It is a common misconception that salt is responsible for many medical problems and for water retention leading to long-term weight gain and cellulite. In fact, extra salt is cleared out of the body within hours. Although you may experience even a 2–3 pound (1–1.3 kg) weight gain the morning after, due to transient water retention, that excess is rapidly lost.

Only the few individuals with kidney disorders, with a particular sensitivity to salt, and some hypertensives must be very careful about how much salt they eat. Apart from those with such problems,

we all require a minimum of 800 mg of sodium each day. Unfortunately we eat an average of 6 to 18 g of salt daily – 8 to 20 times the amount required!

Because salt in food stimulates you to eat more, re-educate your palate. Remove the salt shaker from your kitchen and your table! Savor your food seasoned with other exciting spices like pepper, tarragon, dill, oregano, garlic, onion (not garlic and onion salt), cumin, curry, parsley, sage, rosemary and thyme. It takes about four to eight weeks to adapt to this new, much more interesting way of eating. After that, you will not even like extra salt.

The Unlimited GREFLOF Feast: Fruits and Vegetables

In banishing cellulite, we open for ourselves a whole new world of fabulous cuisine, the world of fruits and vegetables. We can enjoy great meals and feel satisfied and energized, even as our figures become more streamlined. This food is delicious to eat and loaded with the vitamins and minerals we need, but has *no fat*!

As summarized in the table shown on page 61, there are two main categories of carbohydrate: simple carbohydrates (sugars) and complex carbohydrates (starch and fiber). Although all of these give 4 calories for each gram absorbed, you can reduce your cellulite by choosing your carbohydrates wisely.

First, select sugars that will help you. Since fructose (from fruits) is 1.7 times as

59

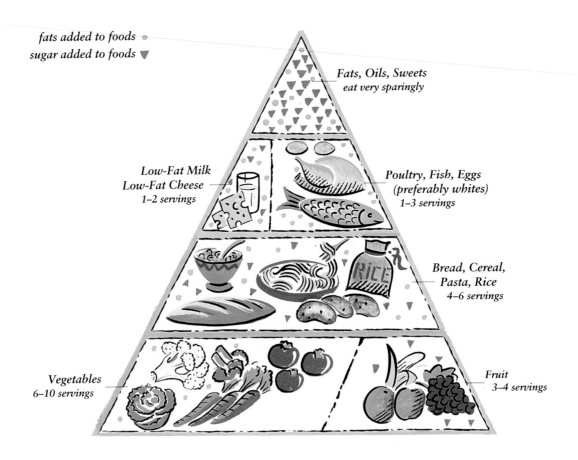

fats added to foods
sugar added to foods

Fats, Oils, Sweets
eat very sparingly

Low-Fat Milk
Low-Fat Cheese
1–2 servings

Poultry, Fish, Eggs
(preferably whites)
1–3 servings

Bread, Cereal,
Pasta, Rice
4–6 servings

Vegetables
6–10 servings

Fruit
3–4 servings

This food pyramid shows recommended daily amounts of different food types.

sweet as sucrose (table sugar), it takes far less fructose to sweeten foods than table sugar – so you get equal sweetness with fewer calories! There are also advantages to the alcohol forms of sugar (which are entirely different from alcohols we drink). These sugar alcohols – mannitol, sorbitol, and xylitol – are not absorbed very quickly, so they cause blood sugar levels to rise slowly. They can therefore be used safely in so-called "diabetic" and "dietetic" foods as well as in sugar-free gums.

Second, favor high-fiber fruits and vegetables which really help you to reduce your cellulite. Fiber is that portion of plants that we can't digest. Soluble fibers attract and hold water in the digestive tract, and insoluble fibers provide bulk to the intestinal contents, delaying stomach emptying. If you wait about 20 minutes after eating fiber, you won't even want a second helping – and you will continue to feel full long after you eat. Furthermore, a large percentage of fiber food is not

60

absorbed – it satiates without staying with you! Unlike starchy foods, which are completely absorbed, less of the weight of high-fiber foods finds its way onto your thighs! Four ounces (125 g) of potato has 70 calories; 4 oz (125 g) of spinach has only 12 calories and broccoli only 25.

What About Sugar?

Sugar is a relatively new addition to our diet. In fact, perhaps the most drastic change in human eating habits in 3 million years is the increased consumption of refined sugar. Sugar did not exist in the times of the Ancient Greeks – there was

CARBOHYDRATES *(Fruits, Vegetables and Grains)*

SIMPLE CARBOHYDRATES (SUGARS)

CLASS	TYPE	FOOD SOURCES	RELATIVE SWEETNESS
Monosaccharides *(simple sugar units)*	Glucose	Fruits, honey, corn syrup	74
	Fructose	Fruits, honey	170
	Galactose	Not found in free foods	16
	Mannitol	Pineapples, olives, asparagus, sweet potatoes, carrots, dietetic products	50
	Sorbitol	Fruits, vegetables, dietetic products	63
	Xylitol	Fruits, vegetables, cereals, mushrooms, seaweed, dietetic gum, dietetic products	90
Disaccharides *(two sugar units)*	Sucrose *(glucose + fructose)*	Sugar cane, sugar beets, maple syrup	100
	Lactose *(glucose + galactose)*	Milk	16
	Maltose *(glucose + fructose)*	Malt products, some breakfast cereals	N/A

COMPLEX CARBOHYDRATES

CLASS	TYPE	FOOD SOURCES
Polysaccharides *(multi-sugars)*	Starch *(easily digestible)*	Wheat, oats, rye, brown rice, vegetables, potatoes, sweet potatoes, green peas, garbanzo beans (chickpeas)
	Fibers Soluble *(pectins and gums)*	Apples, carrots, oats, citrus fruits, legumes, barley
	Insoluble *(cellulose, hemicellulose, lignin)*	Cellulose is found in all plants. Good sources of the insoluble fibers include whole-wheat fiber, bran, edible seeded fruits (like strawberries), fruits and vegetables with edible skins (like apples, pears, peppers)

not even a word for it! Now the average European consumes over 80 pounds (36 kg) of sugar each year – that's 25 teaspoons each day! And the average American eats even more.

Why do sugars have such a bad nutritional reputation? It is not because sugars per se are bad, but because we are moving away from sugar-containing foods to increased use of refined sugars. Instead of getting sugar from fruits and vegetables, we are eating more sugar, combined with highly saturated fats – the Disaster Duo. Furthermore, when we eat concentrated sugars, they are absorbed, raising blood glucose levels. Sugars from whole foods are absorbed more slowly so that the increase in blood glucose is gradual.

As with salt, sugar is added by food manufacturers because they know that sugar increases the amount eaten, and that is good for business. As a result, extra sugar is found in unexpected places – not only in candies, cookies and ice cream, but also in condiments like ketchup and canned fruits and vegetables. The other main culprit is soft drinks: there are six to nine teaspoons of sugar in each 12 fluid ounce (350 ml) can of soda! Each Coke has the sugar equivalent of a piece of chocolate cake with icing. Even popular breakfast cereals are often sugar frosted – with up to 50 percent sugar!

Beware of too much honey! Although honey has been touted as a more natural and presumably healthful sweetener than table sugar or sucrose, it is so concentrated that one teaspoon contains about 21 calories – more than the 15 calories in a teaspoon of sugar. The traces of nutrients in honey have no appreciable value.

My advice is to minimize sugar, particularly sugar plus fat. Try using artificial sweeteners, and drinking only sugar-free beverages or water.

There a number of sugar substitutes available, such as saccharine, the oldest artificial sweetener, and aspartame, (marketed as NutraSweet), which has replaced saccharine as the most widely used artificial sweetener. Only small amounts are needed since aspartame is 180 to 200 times sweeter than sugar.

How to Eat Protein

None of us can live without eating protein. Protein builds our skin, muscle, bone, blood, our organs – everything. The messengers of our bodies (hormones), the mechanisms that run our cells (enzymes), and our protection from foreign attacks (antibodies) – are all proteins and all of these proteins must be constantly replenished. Luckily, most foods contain some protein; only fruits do not contain an appreciable amount. The problem is not in finding enough, but in choosing the best sources and not eating too much.

All protein is made up of 20 building blocks called amino acids. Our bodies can actually make all but nine of these essential acids; the remaining nine must be present in our food. The highest quality proteins contain the essential amino acids proportionate to our needs. Those are from animal sources – egg white, milk, meat and fish. While vegetables and grains are significant sources of the essential amino acids, each one alone often lacks one essential amino acid. Therefore, a person who eats no animal products must learn how to combine. For example, cereals are low in the essential amino acid lysine, while legumes (like peas, beans, and lentils) are low in methionine. A diet containing both rice and beans will have all of the essential amino acids.

How much protein is enough? The current Recommended Daily Allowance for adults is 0.8 grams of protein per kilogram of body weight (about 47 grams of protein per day for a 130-pound/59 kg woman). The amount of protein required decreases with age. Babies require three times as much as adults (relative to their weight).

What are the disadvantages of eating too much protein? Saturated fat and cholesterol accompany animal protein, and nitrogen released in the metabolism of protein must be flushed away by the kidneys, carrying away valuable minerals like calcium, magnesium, and zinc.

High-protein diets (such as the Atkins, Scarsdale, or Stillman diets) are tempting since initial weight-loss is rapid because of the water lost in excreting protein metabolites. However, these diets are not safe long-term, because the body begins to break down its own protein to make the glucose necessary for brain function and energy. Ultimately valuable protein is lost and unwanted fat stays.

I suggest that each day you eat 1-3 portions (weighing 3-4 oz/75-100 g) of protein – preferably an egg-white omelet, chicken or fish, (which have fewer calories than red meat) – and 6-10 portions of fiber vegetables. (All poultry must be cooked without the skin, which contains a lot of fat.) Fish and shellfish are especially low in

GOOD SOURCES OF PROTEIN

	AMOUNT	PROTEIN (g)
Skim milk	1 cup/8 fl oz/250 ml	8
Fish/chicken/ meat	3 oz/75 g	21
Egg white	1	7
Grains		
bread/bagel/	1 slice	3
cereal/pasta rice	½ cup/3 oz/75 g	3
beans/peas lentils	⅓ cup/2 oz/50 g	3
Starchy vegetables		
potatoes	1 small	3
corn	½ cup/3 oz/75 g	3
lima (broad) beans	½ cup/3 oz/75 g	3
Fiber vegetables		
	½ cup/3 oz/75 g *(cooked)*	
asparagus, mushrooms, tomatoes, beets (beetroot), peppers, broccoli, spinach, cabbage, carrots, turnips, eggplant (aubergine), green beans, zucchini (courgette)		2

Recommended daily allowance: 47 g
Cup/imperial/metric conversions are approximate.

fats. If you do choose to eat meat, be sure it is lean – round, sirloin or flank steaks, pork tenderloin, lean veal chops and roasts.

In my GREFLOF Plan I suggest that you do not combine starchy protein with animal protein. This is not an absolute necessity, but does help you eat less. There is no doubt that when you experience many different tastes at one meal, you eat more. Many weight loss diets are based on boredom: eating only rice or fruit not only supplies exclusively a low-calorie food, but also makes you so tired of that one item that you eat only until satiated – or bored; therefore, you end up eating less. The contrast is the "Christmas Dinner Syndrome." You eat the main course of turkey with gravy, potatoes and vegetables until you are absolutely stuffed and you feel you can't eat a bite more. And then the dessert appears and of course you can't resist. If dessert were still more turkey with potatoes, you most certainly wouldn't have one more bite!

Food Combining

Several popular books have been written about "food combining". Their basic philosophy is that the human body cannot digest protein and starch at the same time. Though it is true that starch digestion begins in the mouth with the action of saliva, and protein digestion begins in the stomach, mixing these two does not, in fact, change digestion in any way. There is no physiological evidence that the way

foods are combined alters their ability to be assimilated. However, separating and choosing the types of foods does help psychologically to limit the quantity eaten.

Timing is Everything

The most important rule of eating is, "Eat only when you are hungry, don't eat when you're not hungry!" Luckily, science and the GREFLOF Plan can tell us something about how we can become less hungry.

Medical studies have demonstrated that the rule "Breakfast like a king, lunch like a prince, and dine like a pauper," works for shedding excess fat and cellulite. On one meal a day, you lose more weight if an equal-calorie meal is eaten at 8 a.m. as compared to 5 p.m. Although you do save calories by skipping or having only a minimal breakfast, often eating little after sleeping makes you crave sweets by mid-morning. There is no reason not to have an exciting, low-calorie breakfast. Try a salad or vegetables or, better yet, a protein. A high-protein breakfast tends to depress appetite, while a high-sugar breakfast actually stimulates the appetite!

Eating only once or twice a day causes more weight gain and a greater increase in serum cholesterol than eating the same amount divided over six or more smaller meals. Furthermore, when a diet of 10 or 15 per cent protein is spread over five meals, you lose less total protein than when it is eaten in only one to three sittings. Eating more meals is therefore better for your health and your thighs! So you can enjoy frequent snacks without guilt – as long as they are the right kind.

Vitamins and Minerals That Help You Lose Cellulite

The astonishing fact about vitamins is that small amounts prevent deficiency diseases, but extra supplements markedly improve health. Vitamins, C and E, may directly help to reduce cellulite. Also, as you limit your dairy intake to decrease saturated fats, a calcium supplement is advisable.

Vitamins C and E

It is not possible to get an optimal amount of vitamins C and E from diet alone: you would have to take 44 tablespoons of sunflower oil, equal to 5275 calories of pure fat, and eat more than 100 oranges or many pounds of peppers or blackcurrants to take the amount I recommend.

Vitamins C and E are free-radical quenching antioxidants that protect us against ultraviolet radiation, chemical pollutants, ionizing radiation, thermal burns and many kinds of cancer, strengthen the immune system, and help prevent atherosclerosis, thereby decreasing heart attacks and strokes. If all of these reasons are not enough, the fact that vitamins C and E help fight cellulite most certainly warrants taking them. Both are very important in the remodeling of collagen, especially significant for the structure of cellulite since, as you saw in

Chapter 2, fat cells are packaged in sacs of connective tissue. When our fat cells enlarge (in response to hormones or with weight gain), the connective tissue septae thicken resulting in blood flow being compromised. Vitamin C helps the active remodeling of collagen, and vitamin E alters the cross-linkage of collagen, inhibiting this undesirable thickening. Less thickening equals less cellulite.

Both of these vitamins also protect against possible skin tissue damage. Aerobic exercise generates free radicals with subsequent fat peroxidation which, in turn, damages muscle tissue. The benefits of aerobic exercise, essential for a cellulite-free body, are therefore limited by the formation of lipid peroxides. By quenching free radicals, vitamins C and E help to increase exercise tolerance.

Everyone should take 1000-6000 mg of vitamin C daily, as capsules, effervescent tablets placed in water, or ascorbic acid crystals (1 teaspoon equals 3000 mg) mixed into water or juice.

Most vitamin E on the market is synthetic, a mixture of thirty-two isomers , only one of which (d-α-tocopherol) has significantly higher biological potency. The best form of vitamin E is therefore natural vitamin E – d(not dl)-α-tocopherol, or d-α-tocopheryl acetate (an oil), or d-α-tocopheryl succinate (a dry powder). Everyone should take 400 IU per day (in capsule form) to help live a longer, healthier, and cellulite-free life.

Calcium

Most of us are aware that calcium is of importance to our bones, particularly to prevent osteoporosis in later years. The Recommended Dietary Allowance of calcium for women from 11 to 24 years of age is 1200 mg of calcium per day, from 25 to 60 years 800 mg per day, and from 50 years on 1200 mg per day. Pregnant women should take 1200-1600 mg per day (check with your doctor).

How do we get enough calcium if we limit our intake of dairy products? Since foods with calcium are relatively high in calories, I recommend instead calcium supplements. Calcium citrate, which is better absorbed than calcium carbonate, is best. Supplements such as dolomite and bone meal should be avoided since they may contain lead or other toxic elements. With all these choices, a cellulite-fighter has no excuse not to consume sufficient calcium – it just takes planning.

Alcohol

Alcohol, like sugar, is a nutritional negative because while it provides energy, it is high-calorie with few nutrients. While carbohydrate and protein each provide 4 calories per gram, alcohol yields 7 – almost as much as the 9 calories per gram contributed by fat! Look opposite at the calories some alcoholic drinks contain.

The most negative effect of alcohol involves its metabolism by the liver. When we drink alcohol, it enters the blood and is transported to the liver. There its metabolism is given priority over other foods. Excess alcohol forces the liver to make and store extra fat, causing first a fatty dysfunctional liver and ultimately irreversible liver changes (cirrhosis).

Yet another negative side to alcohol is its effect on control and judgment. We are more likely to indulge in high-fat goodies at a cocktail party after a couple of drinks. And wine with dinner enhances the taste of the food and relaxes us – stimulating us to eat more and to forget all the benefits of the GREFLOF Plan. So limiting alcohol saves calories in more ways than one!

Overall, if you really want to reduce cellulite, I suggest eliminating, or at least minimizing, alcohol.

Dining Out to Reduce Cellulite

Believe it or not, you might find it easier to eat without overindulging when you are not at home because at a restaurant you will not be tempted by seconds, by leftovers, or by the treats that may be in the pantry for your family or roommates.

THE ALCOHOL CALORIE COUNT

Regular beer (12 fl oz/350 ml)	150 cals
Light beer (12 fl oz/350 ml)	95 cals
Gin, rum, vodka, whiskey (2 fl oz/50 ml)	
80 proof	118 cals
90 proof	133 cals
White table wine (6 fl oz/175 ml)	130 cals
Red table wine (6 fl oz/175 ml)	137 cals
Dessert wine (6 fl oz/175 ml)	240 cals
Champagne (6 fl oz/175 ml)	146 cals

The most important thing to keep in mind is not to be shy! You are the customer. If you want to know exactly how a dish is prepared, just ask. There is no difficulty in requesting salad dressings, sauces, and gravy on the side, in having fish, fowl or meat cooked without salt, in having your vegetables non-buttered, in using skim milk instead of whole milk or margarine instead of butter. And it really is so easy to do this subtly.

Try not to go to a restaurant absolutely famished, after not having eaten all day in anticipation. A good hint is to have one of the GREFLOF Happy Hunger Helper snacks (see page 70) before going out, or at least a cup of hot water with lemon. Otherwise, you may stuff yourself with bread and hors d'oeuvres even before ordering! Think before you eat that hot bread so frequently served as soon as you sit down. If it is so truly special, then do have some of it (but without butter, please!). Your philosophy should be not to miss the wonderful special foods, but to limit the quantity and really enjoy what you do eat. If it is just plain bread, wait to start eating until your first course arrives.

When offered drinks before dinner, start with mineral water with lime or a diet soda. (In general try to wait as long as possible in the meal before having alcohol.) On the second round of drinks, have a cocktail or champagne or wine if you wish but try to resist the nibblies as long as possible. Then every second time you wish to reach out for one, sit on your hand. In this way you will enjoy tasting them, but you will eat only half as much!

There are lots of great, low-fat first courses on most menus. You can always order a salad or a vegetable. Do taste any dressing or sauce – but have it served on the side. Instead of pouring it onto your food, dip your fork in the dressing or sauce before eating your food. You will experience the taste with far less.

Select a main course according to the GREFLOF Plan. If you opt for pasta or risotto, have it with vegetables, not meat or fish. If you choose fish or fowl, request an extra order of green vegetables instead of the potatoes or rice. If portions are large, split a main course with a friend or take half home – or order a second appetizer or a salad instead. Don't eat the fatty "decorations" such as olives.

Desserts present a dilemma. Perhaps you can resist the fat plus sugar temptations, having only a special coffee or tea. Fruit is the dessert of choice and can be a wonderful treat. But if there is an extraordinary "Disaster Duo," eat only half and then eat less tomorrow.

What about fast food restaurants? Although these should be avoided, you can often go to the salad bar or have chicken or a plain pizza (and eat only half!) instead of a double cheeseburger or "pepperoni plus" pizza. Maybe there are baked potatoes or corn on the cob. Avoid the onion rings, French fries, and shakes!

67

THE GREFLOF **DAILY PLAN**

BREAKFAST

1. ½ cup/12 fl oz/350 ml unsweetened grapefruit or orange juice

OR

1 serving preferred fruit of your choice

2. Choose one of the following:

(i) Low-calorie bran, blueberry, cranberry, or apple muffin[†]

(ii) Unsweetened cereal (¾ cup/4 oz/125 g preferably of puffed wheat or rice, corn or bran flakes, shredded wheat) with ½ cup /4 fl oz/120 ml non-fat milk

(iii) Egg-white Omelet (see page 71)

(iv) 2-3 Extra-Light Pancakes* (see page 71)

(v) A Super Salad (see page 74)

(vi) 1–3 servings of vegetables

(vii) Rice (hot or cold)[†*] with fruit juice and/or topped with fruit or with cinnamon and artificial sugar syrup.

3. Coffee or tea (with non-fat milk and artificial sweetener if desired)

LUNCH AND DINNER

1. As much green leafy salad or crudités as you wish with no more than 1 tablespoon of low-calorie salad dressing or dip

2a. 1 portion of chicken or fish (a card-deck size which equals about 3 oz/75 g)

OR

½ cup/3 oz/75 g chicken, salmon, or tuna salad on a bed of lettuce

2b. 6 one-quarter sized Special Sandwiches (see page 73)

OR

¾ cup/4 oz/125 g rice or pasta

OR

1 sweet potato or baked white potato with non-fat yogurt and chives or low-calorie dressing or dip

OR

¾ cup/4 oz/125 g garbanzo beans (chickpeas), lima (broad) beans, peas

3. As many green leafy vegetables (cooked without butter, margarine, oil or salt but with any seasoning) as you wish – at least three portions with each meal

4. Coffee or tea (with non-fat milk and artificial sweetener)

[†] *If you wish, add sugar-free jelly or preserves.*

* *If you wish, add artificial sugar syrup.*

NOTES

• **Lunch and dinner**: for both meals choose one item from either **2a** or **2b**. If you choose **2a** for lunch then eat **2b** for dinner. Eat as much of **1** and **3** at each meal as you like.

• Eat one **dessert** other than fruit each day.

• **Do not eat within two hours of retiring at night.** If you are extremely hungry, you may have preferably a diet beverage or tea and/or one apple or ½ grapefruit or any of the Happy Hunger Helpers.

• **To decrease appetite** (especially before a meal)

1. Drink a glass of hot or cold water with the juice of ¼ lemon

2. Eat a green, leafy salad with diet dressing

• **Snacks:** Try one of the Happy Hunger Helpers (see page 70)

VITAMINS

1. Vitamin C: 1000–6000 mg/day

2. Vitamin E: 400 IU/day (d-α-tocopherol,
d-α-tocopheryl succinate or
d-α-tocopheryl acetate)

3. Calcium: 800–1200 mg/day

PREFERRED FRUITS

One serving is equal to:

1 apple, 1 peach or nectarine,
½ cup fresh pineapple,
½ grapefruit or 4 floz/125 ml. unsweetened
grapefruit juice, ½ cup (4oz/125g) blueberries,
strawberries, or raspberries, ½ cantaloupe,
¼ honey dew melon, small slice watermelon.

VEGETABLES

You may eat an unlimited amount of the
following raw or steamed vegetables with
herbal seasoning but no salt, butter or sauce:
asparagus, beets, broccoli, brussels sprouts
cabbage, carrots, cauliflower, celery,
collard greens (spring greens), cucumber,
endive, fennel, green beans, lettuce,
okra, onion, parsley, pea pods,
peppers (red, green or yellow), radish,
spinach, sprouts, squash, tomatoes,
turnips, zucchini (courgette)

ABSOLUTELY FORBIDDEN

• Butter and buttery sauces, all dairy products
except non-fat milk, non-fat yogurt, low-fat
ricotta, cream or cottage cheese, extra salt,
extra sugar, nuts, fatty snacks.

If you absolutely crave sugar:

• Use artificial sweetener

• Eat one serving of fruit

• Drink a diet soda

• Eat a sugar-free hard candy

• Air-pop popcorn and sweeten with artificial
sugar and cinnamon

• Add to cooked rice: fruit and fruit juice or
artificial sugar and cinnamon

• Drink a glass of water with 1 tablespoon
lemon juice or 1 tablespoon cider vinegar and
artificial sweetener (this drink is really
refreshing hot or cold; with vinegar, it tastes
like apple cider).

THE GREFLOF RULES

*By following only a few simple rules, you can
become healthier, energized, and cellulite free –
and you may very well live longer to enjoy all this!*

1. Fat is Fattening
   • eat less than about 35 grams per day
   • avoid all fat and sugar combinations
   • avoid fat and salt combinations
   • avoid saturated (animal) fat
   • use only unsaturated (vegetable) oils.
2. Feast on fruits and vegetables
3. Avoid any extra sugar; use artificial
   sweeteners instead
4. Eat the right kind of protein, but not too
   much of it
5. Eat more frequent, smaller meals and eat
   your larger meals earlier in the day
6. Each day, take
   vitamin C (ascorbic acid):   1000–6000 mg
   vitamin E (d-α-tocopherol): 400 IU
   calcium: 800–1200 mg
7. Minimize alcohol
8. Don't go out to eat starving, and don't be
   shy about ordering what you want

HAPPY HUNGER HELPERS

1. Carrot and celery sticks. Store standing in a glass in the refrigerator with a little water in the bottom or carry to work in a zip–lock plastic bag after washing without drying
2. Cut slices of:
red, yellow or green pepper, cucumber, cherry tomatoes, lettuce leaves
3. Air-popped popcorn made with seasonings, with no butter or salt. If you must add butter, use low-calorie, low-fat types. Try seasonings such as cumin, cinnamon with artificial sweetener, curry, onion, garlic, dill, cilantro (coriander), sage, thyme
4. Seltzer water mixed with grapefruit, orange, pineapple, apple or cranberry juice
5. Hot or cold water with a slice of lemon, lime, or orange, or with a tablespoon of cider vinegar and artificial sweetener
6. Half an apple or any portion of the preferred fruits listed on page 69
7. Low-calorie hard candies.
8. Rice cakes, wheat cakes
9. Non-sweetened cereals: especially puffed wheat and puffed rice, corn flakes, bran flakes, shredded wheat

COOKING TIPS

1. You can create your own low-calorie, low-fat dishes from favorite recipes by seasoning without salt and by astute substitutions.

Substitute:
ground pepper, chopped garlic
dill, coriander, grated ginger
for *salt*

dried beans and lentils
for *meat in casseroles and stews*

poultry
for *meat in meatloaf, chilli and steaks*

non-fat yogurt
for *sour cream, mayonnaise in salads*

cornstarch (cornflour) or arrowroot
for *flour as a thickener*

spaghetti squash
for *spaghetti*

grated carrots or celery
for *breadcrumbs*

chicken broth
for *butter or oil to sauté*

2. Always remove skin from poultry and fish before cooking
3. Always remove all visible fat from meats, poultry and fish before cooking
4. Always use non-stick cookware (with spray of no-calorie, no-fat vegetable oil when necessary) instead of butter or oil for frying and sautéing
5. Cook mushrooms, tomatoes, green peppers and other vegetables in the microwave for 2 minutes, covered, with a few drops of water in the pan
6. Don't ever add breadcrumbs to ground (minced) beef or poultry. They soak in the fat rather than let it drip off.
7. Make croûtons for soups and salads from whole grain light bread in the microwave or toaster *without* adding any butter or margarine

BREAKFAST

There is no reason why breakfast has to be the same day in and day out – try rice, a salad or vegetables for a change. Breakfast can be the most exciting and variable meal of the day! Why not try out some of these smashing ideas and see for yourself!

EXTRA–LIGHT PANCAKES

Makes 8 pancakes
1 pancake: 81 cals • fat 0 g

1 cup /8 fl oz/250 ml pancake mix
½ cup /4 fl oz/120 ml skim milk
2 egg whites
juice of ½ an orange

1) Mix all the ingredients with a wire whisk until well blended.
2) Pour ¼ cup/2 fl oz/50 ml of the mixture onto a hot, non–stick frying pan (skillet).
3) Cook until the edges are dry. Turn and cook until golden.

EGG–WHITE OMELET

Serves 1 • cals: 68 • fat: 0 g

2 egg whites
1 tablespoon non-fat milk
1 tablespoon chopped parsley
chopped or grated vegetables

1) Beat the egg whites with 1 tablespoon of non-fat milk or water. (Egg whites are best beaten when at room temperature.)
2) Season the eggs with parsley and pepper.

3) Pour into a hot non-stick frying pan. Cook on a low flame until the edges are almost dry.
4) Next top with any combination of chopped or grated vegetables you like, such as tomato, red or green peppers, mushrooms, onions, and carrots.
5) Fold and turn. Cook until light brown.

APPLE BRAN MUFFINS

Makes 12 • 1 muffin: 112 cals • fat: 0.9 g

½ cup /4 fl oz/120 ml water
½ cup/2 oz/50 g powdered milk
3 eggs, beaten
2 apples, chopped with skin
1 teaspoon cinnamon
¼ teaspoon nutmeg
½ teaspoon vanilla extract
1 teaspoon baking powder
1 teaspoon baking soda
artificial sweetener to taste
2 cups/12 oz/350g unprocessed bran

1) Mix together all the ingredients except the bran. Stir until thoroughly mixed. (Do not use a blender.)
2) Stir in the unprocessed bran.
3) Pour the mixture into muffin cups lined with paper baking cups.
4) Bake in a preheated oven at 350°F/180°C/Gas Mark 4 for 25–30 minutes (until no longer moist when pierced with a knife or toothpick).
5) Cool, then refrigerate until served.

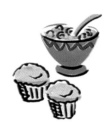

SUPER SALADS AND SANDWICHES

Salads are the most important foods for attaining and maintaining a cellulite-free body. Low in calories and fat, high in fiber, rich with vitamins and minerals, salads are very healthy. Salads are easy: keep washed lettuce, spinach, or endive (chicory) in the refrigerator covered with a damp paper towel. Crudités can be precut and refrigerated in a little water. You can make large quantities of the salad dressing recipes to refrigerate for up to 1 or 2 months.

ENDIVE SALAD

Serves 4 • 1 tbs: 53 cals • 5.2 g fat

2 endives (heads of chicory)
1 bunch watercress, chopped
1 tablespoon Lemon-Dijon Vinaigrette

1) Wash and slice the endives (chicory).
2) Mix with the watercress.
3) Add the Lemon–Dijon Vinaigrette. Place portions directly on salad plates for an elegant first course or for a side salad.

LEMON–DIJON VINAIGRETTE

1 tbs: 48 cals • 5.2 g fat

3 tablespoons vegetable oil
4 tablespoons lemon juice
2 teaspoons Dijon mustard
½ teaspoon black pepper

1) Put all ingredients into a jar and shake.
2) Use on salads or as a dip for crudités.

COLE SLAW

Serves 8 • 1 serving: 25 cals • 1.3 g fat

1 medium head of white cabbage, chopped
1 onion, chopped
1 cup/6 oz/175 g chopped celery
1 green pepper, cut in strips
1 teaspoon salt
dash of paprika
1 teaspoon celery seed
1 teaspoon white mustard seed
½ cup /4 fl oz/120 ml apple cider vinegar
artificial sweetener to taste
2 teaspoons diet mayonnaise or vegetable oil

1) Mix together the cabbage, onion, celery and green pepper.
2) In a separate bowl, mix the remaining ingredients. Pour over cabbage and mix thoroughly.
3) Chill for 6 hours.
4) Before serving, add the diet mayonnaise or vegetable oil and sprinkle with paprika.

TART VINAIGRETTE

1 tbs: 36 cals • 3.9 g fat

¼ cup /2 fl oz/50 ml extra virgin oil
⅔ cup/5 1/2 fl oz/165 ml red wine vinegar
1 clove garlic
1/2 teaspoon dried oregano
1 anchovy, finely chopped or puréed (optional)
black pepper to taste

1) Combine all ingredients in a jar and shake.

DILL CHICKEN OR SALMON SALAD

Serves 4 • 1 serving: 132 cals • 5.1 g fat

2 baked or boiled chicken breasts cut in cubes or
12 oz/350 g salmon, canned in water
¼ cup/1 tablespoon fresh chopped dill
freshly ground pepper to taste
To garnish: sliced cucumber
celery sticks
sliced or cherry tomatoes

1) Mix the ingredients and place on a
generous bed of lettuce.
2) Garnish with sliced vegetables.

SUPER TOFU SPICE DIP

Serves 4 • 1 tbs: 62 cals • fat: 0 g

8 oz/225 g pressed tofu
onion powder, garlic powder, mustard (to taste)
2 tablespoons finely chopped red pepper
2 tablespoons finely chopped green pepper

1) Mash the tofu.
2) Mix the tofu with all the other ingredients.
Serve with crudités or with diet crackers.

Try the following variations:
Curry dip: Add 1 teaspoon curry powder
Onion dip: Add 2 teaspoons chopped onion
plus chopped scallions (spring onions).
Garlic dip: Add 2 pressed or chopped fresh
garlic cloves
Chive dip: Add 1 tablespoon chives

SUPER GREEN SPINACH SAUCE

1 tbs: 7 cals • 0.1 g fat

1 lb/450 g fresh spinach
½ cup /4 fl oz/120 ml chicken broth
1 scallion (spring onion)
1 tablespoon fresh cilantro (coriander)
¼ teaspoon pepper
few drops of lemon juice

1) Cook the spinach in boiling chicken broth
for 3–4 minutes.
2) Place in a blender and add all the other
ingredients. Blend to a smooth purée.

SPECIAL SANDWICHES

¼ sandwich: 40 cals • 1 g fat

These are great for lunch or tea or dinner!
Use thin sliced, low-calorie ("light") whole
grain or whole wheat (wholemeal) bread.
These sandwiches are excellent dry with no
mayonnaise, but you may add a minimal
amount (½–1 teaspoon per slice of bread) of
diet mayonnaise to the bread. This adds
approximately 15 cals per quarter sandwich.
Fill the sandwiches generously with slices of
tomato, chopped lettuce, chopped egg white,
green pepper, watercress and cucumber.
Trim the bread crusts, and cut each sandwich
diagonally into quarters.
Arrange decoratively,
alternating the colors, and
garnish with sprigs of parsley
or coriander.

73

MAIN COURSES

Chicken is lower in fat and calories than other meats, and turkey is even lower. A portion is 3 oz/75 g. A great method of cooking fish or fowl is "en papillote." Place the chicken or fish on a piece of baking parchment, add herbs and lemon juice (and a dab of tomato sauce, if you wish), fold and bake at 350°F/180°C/Gas Mark 4 for 40 minutes. The parchment seals in the juices.

A quick, lively, and unusual sauce for chicken or fish can be made with a purée of 3 red peppers blended with 3 tablespoons of chicken stock.

The **Super Green Spinach Sauce** on page 73 is also excellent with chicken.

CHICKEN BREASTS FLORENTINE

Serves 4 • 1 serving: 116 cals • fat: 4.2 g

2 cups/6 oz/175 g fresh spinach (1 package)
¼ cup/2 oz/50 g onion slices
2 x 4-oz/100-g chicken breast, cut in half
garlic, pepper, onion powder
1 tablespoon apple cider vinegar

1) Place the spinach leaves on a large piece of tin foil and top with the onion slices.
2) Lay half a chicken breast per person on the bed of spinach.
3) Season with pepper, garlic or onion powder to taste, then sprinkle with a little cider vinegar.
4) Fold the foil into a pouch. Cook in a preheated oven at 350°F/180°C/Gas Mark 4 for 25-30 minutes.

SEAFOOD ON SKEWERS

Serves 4 • 1 serving: 130 cals • fat: 6.6g

3 oz/75 g each of 3 types of fish, cut into 1-inch/2.5-cm cubes: halibut, swordfish, shrimp, scallops, salmon, monkfish
cherry tomatoes; onions, cut in quarters; green and red peppers, cut into chunks

Marinade:
juice of 1 lemon
2 tablespoons onion powder
2 tablespoons balsamic vinegar
1 clove garlic, crushed
1 envelope instant chicken broth

1) Marinate the fish for about 1-2 hours.
2) Thread the fish and vegetables alternately onto wooden or metal skewers.
3) Broil (grill) for about 10-15 minutes until light brown.

LIME–BROILED CHICKEN

Serves 4 • 1 serving: 196 cals • fat: 10 g

Lime barbecue sauce:
4 skinless chicken breasts
1 tablespoon corn oil
4 tablespoons lime juice
1 teaspoon dried tarragon
½ teaspoon salt
½ teaspoon tabasco

1) Mix ingredients and brush on chicken.
2) Broil (grill) for about 10-15 minutes.

FLOUNDER (PLAICE) IN LETTUCE POUCHES

Serves 4 • 1 serving: 80 cals • fat: 11 g

4 lettuce leaves, rinsed
¼ cup minced chives
1 tablespoon fresh dill or 1 teaspoon dried dill
¼ teaspoon pepper
2 teaspoons mustard
2 x 8-oz/225 g flounder (plaice) fillets (or swordfish, halibut, salmon, red snapper, or sole)

1) Microwave the lettuce leaves on High for 1 minute in a 1½–quart/2 ¼ pt/⅓ litre casserole (covered with plastic wrap with one corner open to vent), or steam until soft. Drain the lettuce on paper towels.
2) Mix the seasonings together.
3) Split the fish fillets lengthwise. Spread the seasonings evenly over each fillet.
4) Roll up each fillet of fish in a lettuce leaf, beginning with the short end, and place carefully in the casserole.
5) Cover with heavy-duty plastic wrap with one corner open to vent. Microwave on High for 4–5 minutes or bake covered in a preheated oven at 400°F/200°C/Gas Mark 6 for 20–25 minutes.

Note

When making any of the recipes in this book follow only one set of measurements as they are not interchangeable.

PASTA PRIMAVERA

Serves 4 • 1 serving: 341 cals • fat: 11g

Pasta:

8-10 oz/225-300 g spaghetti, angel hair pasta, capellini or penne
1 teaspoon olive oil

Primavera:

1 cup/4 oz/125 g broccoli spears
1 cup/6 oz/175 g pea pods
2 teaspoons olive oil
4-5 cloves garlic, crushed
6 cherry tomatoes
1 green pepper, cut into large cubes
1 red pepper, cut into large cubes
1 bunch arugula (rocket), cut
12-15 leaves fresh basil
grated low-fat parmesan cheese (optional)

1) Cook the pasta of your choice according to the package instructions, adding a teaspoon of olive oil to the water.
2) Steam the broccoli for 2–3 minutes
3) Blanch the pea pods quickly in boiling water for 1 minute.
4) Heat the olive oil and garlic in a pan. Add the cherry tomatoes, green pepper, red pepper, and arugula (rocket) and cook for 2 minutes, stirring continuously.
5) Add the vegetables (and basil) to the pasta and toss.
6) If you wish, top with a sprinkling of grated low-fat parmesan cheese.

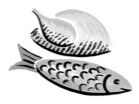

VEGETABLES

Vegetables are delicious steamed only lightly so that they remain crunchy. This leaves not only the taste but also the nutrients.

Try different vegetables such as fennel, okra, spaghetti squash, turnips, and zucchini (courgette). Enhance the flavor with exciting spices such as tarragon, caraway seeds, garlic, paprika, basil, marjoram, dill, thyme, parsley, oregano and balsamic vinegar or lemon juice. Do not add salt! For a true energy boost, drink the water that remains after steaming – either hot (immediately after cooking) or cold.

It is especially important to purchase your vegetables carefully. Believe it or not, the most nutritious vegetables are frozen ones, since the best of each crop is chosen immediately after picking for freezing. Once frozen, the nutrients are preserved. Choose the vegetables that seem the most plentiful and the least expensive. They are usually the freshest, since they may have been grown locally. (One–third of the cost of any vegetable is the cost of transport.)

TERRIFIC TURNIPS

Serves 6 • 1 serving: 20 cals • fat: 0.1 g

5 turnips
½ large potato
dash of cayenne pepper

1) Steam the turnips and potato.
2) Mash with a potato masher or purée in a food processor.

ARTICHOKES WITH GARLIC

Serves 2 • 1 serving (without dressing):
65 cals • fat: 0.2g

2 artichokes
1 cup/8 fl oz/250 ml boiling water
1 clove garlic, chopped
1 slice of lemon
Lemon–Dijon Vinaigrette, to serve

1) Cut the artichokes at the base. Trim, discarding the thicker lower leaves.
2) Place in a covered saucepan with the boiling water, garlic and lemon. Simmer for 30–40 minutes until soft.
3) Place on a plate. Remove some of the leaves from the center top to arrange decoratively around the base.
4) Serve hot with Lemon-Dijon Vinaigrette.

FRESH POTATO CHIPS

1 serving: 60 cals • fat 2.5 g

1 large potato
white vinegar
chopped chives or dill to taste

1) Cut 1 large peeled potato into about 20 thin slices.
2) Spread on a non-stick cookie (biscuit) tray, or pre-sprayed with non-fat cooking spray.
3) Broil (grill) for 4 minutes at medium heat.
4) Turn; bake on other side for 4 minutes.
5) Sprinkle with white vinegar and dill, chives or other preferred herbs.

PEPPER TRICOLORE

Serves 6 • 1 serving: 35 cals • fat: 1.0 g

1 tablespoon water
1 teaspoon vegetable oil
2 green peppers, cored, deseeded and cut
into strips
1 red pepper, cored, deseeded and cut into strips
1 yellow pepper, cut into strips
1 clove garlic, crushed
¼ dried whole oregano
2 tablespoons vinegar

1) In a large skillet (frying pan) coated with non–fat cooking spray, heat the water and oil.
2) Add the peppers, garlic, and oregano. Sauté for 3 minutes, stirring constantly.
3) Remove from the heat and stir in vinegar.

SPINACH ZUCCHINI HARMONY

Serves 6 • 1 serving: 35 cals • 2.5 g fat

1 zucchini (courgette) with skin
1 teaspoon olive oil
1 clove garlic, chopped
1 lb/450 g spinach
½ cup /4 fl oz/120 ml chicken broth

1) Wash the zucchini (courgette), scrubbing with a brush. Grate with a cheese grater
2) Heat the olive oil with the garlic. Sauté the zucchini (courgette) in a non-stick skillet (frying pan).
3) Cook the spinach in boiling chicken broth for 5 minutes. Mix with the zucchini.

RATATOUILLE

Serves 6 • 1 serving: 60 cals • fat: 2.5 g

½ tablespoon olive oil
1 large onion, finely chopped
1 garlic clove, crushed with ½ teaspoon salt
1 lb/450 g zucchini (courgette), sliced
1 lb/450 g tomatoes, skinned, seeded and chopped or 1 x 14–oz/400 g can tomatoes
1 large eggplant (aubergine), sliced and peeled
1 green pepper, cored, seeded and sliced
freshly ground black pepper
¼ teaspoon thyme
¼ teaspoon oregano

1) Heat the olive oil in a large saucepan. Add the onion and garlic and fry together until golden brown.
2) Add all the remaining chopped vegetables to the saucepan. Season with pepper, thyme and oregano (or any other herb flavorings you like) and add enough water to come about halfway up the vegetables.
3) Bring the mixture to a boil, stirring constantly, then lower the heat, cover and simmer gently for about 30 minutes, stirring occasionally. The vegetables should be soft and the juices thick.
4) Season to taste and transfer to a hot serving dish. Alternatively cool and chill in the refrigerator and eat as a salad with lettuce.
5) Before serving sprinkle with parsley.

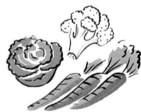

DESSERTS

The very best dessert is fresh fruit, which can be presented like a work of art. Sliced melon topped with lemon and a mint leaf, mixed berries, orange slices (sprinkled with Grand Marnier for special occasions), pineapple decorated with raspberries or strawberries all satisfy your sweet tooth and end a meal with pizzazz. Here are some other great dessert recipes for you to try.

BLUSHING PEARS

Serves 4 • 1 serving: 145 cals • fat: 0.7 g

4 pears, peeled
juice of ½ lemon
1 orange, sliced, with rind

Raspberry sauce:
1 package (12 oz/350 g) frozen or fresh
*   raspberries*
1½ teaspoons artificial sweetener

1) Cover the pears with water in a large saucepan. Add lemon juice and sliced oranges.
2) Simmer for 20–25 minutes. Check that they are soft by piercing with a fork.
3) Stand on a plate with raspberries or strawberries and top with a mint leaf.
4) Purée the raspberries in a blender with artificial sweetener.
5) Strain through a fine strainer to remove all the seeds.
6) Pour a little of the raspberry sauce on to the pears before serving and serve in a sauceboat on the side.

ANGEL FOOD CAKE

Serves 12 • 1 serving: 48 cals • fat: 0 g

6 egg whites
½ teaspoon cream of tartar
⅛ teaspoon salt
¼ cup plus 2 tablespoons/3 oz/75 g sugar
½ cup/2 oz/50 g sifted cake (self–raising) flour
½ teaspoon vanilla extract
¼ teaspoon orange extract

1) Beat egg whites until foamy. Add cream of tartar and salt. Beat until soft peaks form.
2) Gradually add the sugar, 2 tablespoons at a time, beating until stiff peaks form.
3) Sprinkle the flour over the mixture.
4) Pour the batter into an ungreased 9-inch/23-cm round cake pan (tin).
5) Bake in a preheated oven at 325°F/170°C/Gas Mark 3 for 30 minutes (until a knife inserted comes out clean).
6) Cool in the pan (tin) for 40 minutes.

COFFEE GRANITA

Serves 4 • 1 serving: 25 cals • fat: 0 g

1) Mix 1 cup of espresso coffee with 1 cup of instant coffee. Add artificial sweetener to taste. Place in container in freezer.
2) When the surface hardens remove and chop. Repeat process several times until a texture of well-crushed ice is achieved.

HINTS TO HELP YOU BE THE WEIGHT YOU WANT TO BE

1) Socialize with friends at places where you do not eat. Walk in the park or window shop.

2) Never go food shopping hungry.

3) Slow down! Always eat sitting down, actively savoring every bite as you chew.

4) Designate a specific place to eat at home or at work. This will help you break the habit of eating on the run.

5) Never eat in front of television, at the movies, or as a spectator watching sports. This will break any habitual, innocuous eating. And if you do snack, eat Happy Hunger Helpers.

6) Eat only when you are hungry!

7) Cut your food into small pieces; take small bites; chew each bite at least 10 times.

8) If you are served a large portion in a restaurant, simply decide immediately to eat only half. Divide your food into this half-portion as soon as the plate is placed in front of you.

9) Order appetizers as main courses.

10) Try to eat slower than everyone else.

11) Taste your food! Don't add extra salt, especially without tasting first.

12) Fill salt shakers with other seasonings.

13) When eating in restaurants, always specify that any sauces, sour cream, butter, margarine, and salad dressings be served "on the side," so that you control exactly the extra fat you eat.

14) Try salads without dressing – or with lemon or balsamic vinegar and herbs only.

15) Always keep Happy Hunger Helpers nearby and ready for snack attacks!

16) Fry in non-stick pans with low-calorie, non-fat cooking spray instead of butter or oil.

17) Always remove the skin and fat from chicken and fish before cooking.

18) Never, never, never eat between snacks!

19) Any time you are hungry between meals, delay. Wait 20 minutes: do some Pressometrics or read an article. You will probably not even be hungry any more (a scientifically proven fact!)

20) If you are still hungry after a 20–minute delay, drink a large glass of hot or cold water (flavored with lemon or lime or orange), then wait 20 minutes more. If you are still hungry, eat a Happy Hunger Helper.

21) If you do have a particular food craving, first follow rules 19 and 20. If you still absolutely must eat that food, allow yourself three small bites. Throw the rest away, *even before you eat.* Do not let one moment of breaking your eating plan become an excuse to binge

22) If you live alone, throw out all the fatty junk food you have immediately! If your family or roommate absolutely must eat fattening foods, then keep them all in a separate place.

23) Avoid buffets! If you must go, use a salad or dessert plate instead of a large dinner plate – or better yet, a saucer! (The so-called Saucer Diet is to eat no more than will fit on a saucer at each meal!)

24) If you are a nervous nibbler, chew sugar–free gum instead of munching food.

25) Remember food from other people's plates has calories too, and so do leftovers!

26) Eat only foods you like! Do not eat just to be polite. It is better to throw away those calories than have them stored on your hips!

27) Never go out hungry, especially for lunch, cocktails or dinner!

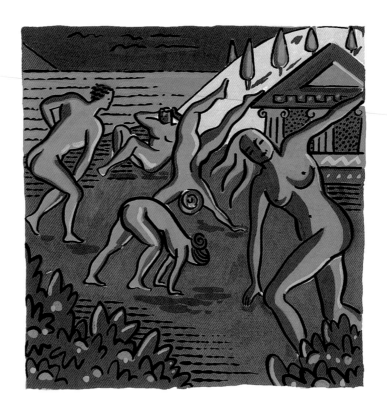

A better body in minutes a day

We all have excuses as to why we don't exercise regularly, but none of them is good enough to explain why we cannot take a few minutes each day to take care of the only thing that is truly ours in life – our bodies. We owe it to ourselves to keep our bodies in good form, to maintain our flexibility and range of motion, and to do all we can to help our body function to its full potential.

No matter how out of shape we are, we *can* get into shape in a relatively short time. It took years for that unattractive, lumpy, bumpy cellulite to form on our hips and thighs; we can eliminate it in weeks with the commitment of only minutes each day and the joy of three or four exercise sessions each week.

Life is change! Each day our body is rebuilding itself: new cells are formed, new tissue is synthesized. Our red blood cells renew themselves every four months; our skin forms a new layer of cells each day; our bones are always in the process of restructuring themselves. If we can recover from even drastic injury to our bodies (after accidents or surgery), we can certainly recover from the consequences of years of poor diet and non-optimal posture and movement. And the way we recover through exercise is not work; it's *fun*! It is a luxury to take even a short time for yourself, to feel the working of your own body, to delight as you see improvement each day. You will be more comfortable with your body; you will carry yourself with pride; you will no longer waste energy worrying about how you look, because you will have taken action and the results will show.

The toughest part of exercising is taking the first step. The thought of going to a gym or exercise class among fit people is intimidating, especially if you feel unathletic and are self-conscious about cellulite. With my exercise routine you will learn, and your body will improve in the privacy of your own home. Your body resculpting can be accomplished with this easy, three-part plan:

1. The *Pressometric* isometric movements, which can be done anywhere, anytime to give your thighs, buttocks and arms a svelte line.

2. The *Twelve-Minute Miracle* daily exercise routine is designed to resculpt cellulite-laden areas. These subtle, controlled, non-strenuous movements preceded by the *Streamline Stretches* are based on yoga and ballet.

3. Your own individual *aerobic exercises* that you will really enjoy doing three or four times each week. You can walk in pretty or interesting places; you can go dancing; you can skip rope; you can just move to music. You might join a gym to use exercise equipment, or to take calisthenics classes, or swim; you might buy a bicycle or a home exercise machine. But you need not go to all that expense. All you really need to accomplish your own aerobics is a good pair of shoes and the commitment to exercise regularly.

To be truly health-giving, exercise must become a permanent pattern in your life. It is as important for maintaining your vitality as food. Movement preserves youth; if you do not move and stretch enough, your body ages prematurely. Your routine must therefore be an enjoyable and convenient treat, so you will not be tempted to put it off for another day.

POSTURE

Do you want to look thinner instantly? You can, simply by standing with better posture! And good posture also eliminates unnecessary aches and improves breathing.

Just stand in front of the mirror in a bathing suit or leotard, facing sideways. Contract your buttocks and tuck in your stomach in the Hip Hugger (see page 85). You will immediately appear thinner. This contracted position also corrects any exaggerated inward curvature of the lower back. This is important, especially if you frequently wear high heels, which can increase "lumbar lordosis" causing an unattractive protrusion of both the stomach and the buttocks.

Now use a second mirror to look at your rear view. As you tighten your buttocks in the Hip Hugger, you see that the sides of your thighs have a smoother line, your buttocks move up, and you look like the "after" of surgical liposuction – all from just standing straight with an isometric pelvic contraction.

The secret of good posture is simply to sit, stand and walk *tall*. To achieve this without straining your body by pushing yourself into the "shoulders back" posture just pretend you are suspended like a puppet by one string from the top of your head. This image automatically causes you to straighten your neck, shoulders, and back without artificial contortion. Your shoulders are relaxed and your chest is naturally lifted.

Just look at these photographs to see how much better you look when you sit up straight. Using the image of being suspended by a string helps you not only to keep your back and shoulders straight without neck and back discomfort, but also to distribute your weight evenly on your pelvic bones when you sit. If you habitually lean to one side as you sit (photograph below), eventually you will stretch the muscles on one side of your body and contract those on the other side, resulting in an actual s-shaped curvature of the spine called scoliosis. This curvature will then affect your posture when you are standing and walking as well.

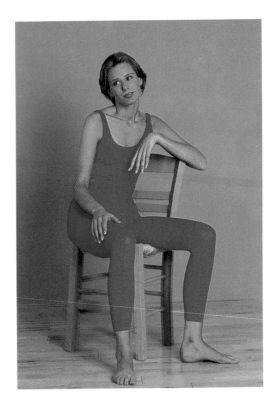

Don't ignore the importance of good posture when sitting. Most of us sit from 8 to 14 hours each day – in the office, in the car, in front of the TV. We spend most of our day moving from chair to sofa to seat. Just look at the photographs below to see how dramatically thinner your hips and waist appear when you sit straight.

WHATEVER SHALL I WEAR?

Women are so lucky! Not only can we change from looking tired and bedraggled to appearing fresh and energetic by applying a little makeup, but we have a great range of diversity in what we can wear. Our clothes can uplift our mood.

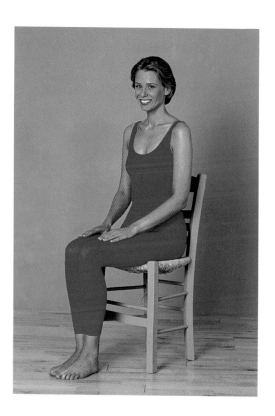

A great outfit for an exercise can actually motivate us to do it!

Your exercise clothes should have three main features:

1. They should be comfortable, so that you can stretch and move. Your clothes should not be constrictive or itchy! Cotton is probably the best fabric since it allows sweat to evaporate.

2. They should be in flattering colors.

3. They should be easily washed, so that you don't avoid vigorous exercise for fear of perspiring (not that all exercise requires sweat for gain!).

You can conceal your flaws by choosing your clothes wisely. Cover flabby arms or thighs with baggy tee shirts or sweatsuits. If you have a bottom-heavy figure, loose tops over leotards, tights or leggings are flattering. Leotards in monochromatic darker colors do make you appear slimmer, especially if they have long sleeves and turtlenecks or "V" necks. To camouflage a bulging stomach leotards should be firm, with vertical side stripes or a "V" pattern or inset. Belts and leotards with thongs can be uncomfortable and restrictive. Leotards cut high at the hips make upper thighs and buttocks appear slimmer and sagging bottoms higher.

You must also be sure to pick the right shoes, ones with good structural support and cushioned soles to absorb impact, especially for walking or running. It is best to buy your shoes late in the day when your feet may be slightly swollen.

PRESSOMETRICS

If I told you that you could truly achieve a more svelte line to your thighs and buttocks within four weeks, that you could achieve this without taking time from your routine activities and that you would require no expensive equipment to accomplish this remarkable feat, wouldn't you definitely want to learn how? There is no excuse for anyone *not* to!

These exercises are for women who want shapely thighs but who hate "exercise." The movements are not boring, nor hard work. They do not tire you; rather they energize you. They are fun; they give you a healthy glow, improved posture, and elegance in movement. Ultimately you will radiate self-confidence because of your visible improvement.

The advantage of these Pressometrics is that you can do them any time. You incorporate these carefully controlled subtle movements into your daily activities. As you brush your teeth and shower in the morning, you can do the Hip Hugger. As you brew your coffee you can do the Latin Lover Leg Lift. As you wait for the elevator or bus you can do Elevator Wait Lift. Working at your desk or watching television, you can do the Ball Crusher and the Saddle Battle. In any bus, train, plane or car you can go into Suspended Animotion or the Kneecap Kiss. Anytime you walk, you can "walk tight" with the Hip Hugger. With Pressometrics even boring activities (such

as tiresome meetings, or standing in line or waiting for appointments) become fun. You can become happy and energized by challenging yourself to do each movement for a longer count than you had achieved the previous occasion. These movements will become second nature to you, a permanent part of your life – and so will your new svelte silhouette!

Since you can do these exercises virtually anywhere, you can incorporate repetitions of any of the Pressometrics into your day without using any extra time and without anyone knowing what you are up to.

The Hip Hugger is one of the simplest and most effective exercises you can learn. It accomplishes both tightening and strengthening simultaneously. Your thighs and buttocks will become firmer; your abdominal muscles stronger, your stomach flatter. You will also strengthen your lower back muscles to improve posture and protect against back strain.

■ Pressometric Tips

1. Initially hold each contraction for a count of 10. Gradually work your way up to a count of 30.

2. Start with three repetitions of each contraction. Increase gradually to 10 repetitions at a time.

3. Increase the number of sets you do each day, especially those that act on your particular trouble spots.

4. Think about the muscles as you contract.

▼ **Hip Hugger** *The Hip Hugger, also known as the Pelvic Tuck, is the easiest and most effective exercise for toning your thighs and buttocks. Stand with your feet shoulder width apart and your hands on your hips (**1**). Contract your abdominal muscles, and squeeze your buttocks together (hard!). Your pelvis will move forward so that you look thinner and more toned instantly (**2**). You will also feel the squeeze in your outer and inner thighs. Pretend you are grasping a pencil between your buttocks, or a thin piece of paper between your thighs. Hold this contraction initially for a count of 10, and work your way up to a count of 30.*

The Hip Hugger is possibly the single most effective "cellulite burner."

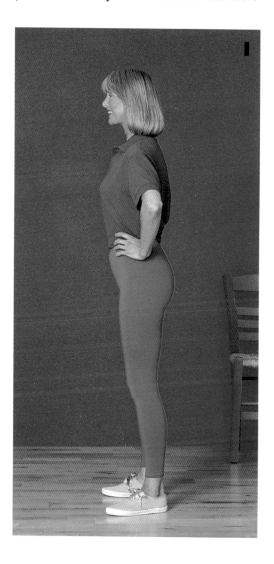

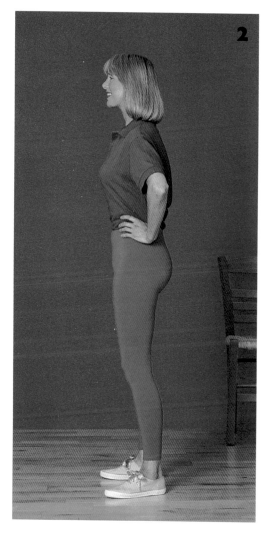

▼ **The Saddle Battle** *Sit forward on a hard chair without arms, closer to the right corner of the chair. With straight arms, grasp the bottom or back of the chair on each side. Place your left foot flat in front of the chair, somewhat towards the right side. Lift your right leg back along the right side of the chair with your knee bent so that your lower leg is parallel to the side of the chair. Keeping your back straight, tuck your pelvis forward and think of pointing your knee into the floor while raising your foot to the ceiling. Now move your right knee gently back about three inches (7.5 cm); hold for a count of ten, then return to the initial position. The movement is quite small; it should be done smoothly. Repeat three times. Position yourself close to the left front corner of the chair and repeat for the left leg.*

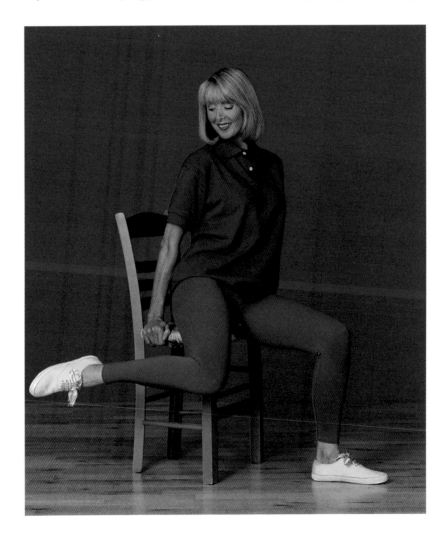

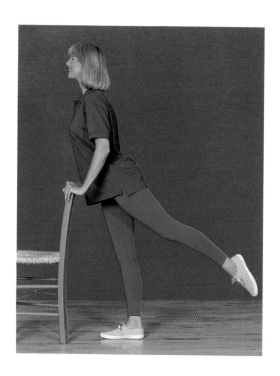

◄ **Latin Lover Leg Lift** *Stand straight, preferably with one hand on a support such as a wall or chair. Lift your left leg back and to the side, raising your foot about four inches (10 cm) from the ground with your toe pointed. Be consciously aware of the contraction of both your front and back thigh muscles. Hold for a count of 10. Repeat at least three times, first with your toe pointed, then with your foot flexed; and then do the same with your right leg.*
VARIATION: *Move the raised leg upwards and downwards almost imperceptibly, the toes alternately pointed then flexed.*

▶ **The Ball Crusher** *Because it is squeezable, a child's ball is best to use, preferably about four to six inches (10–15 cm) in diameter – just keep it near the places you sit. Sit up straight at the edge of your chair. With your feet together, place the ball between your knees and keep it in place by applying pressure with your inner thighs. Squeeze the ball as hard as you can, feeling the contraction of your inner thighs. Hold for a count of 10, then relax, but keep the ball in place. Repeat at least three times. This is the one best exercise you can do for your inner thighs.*

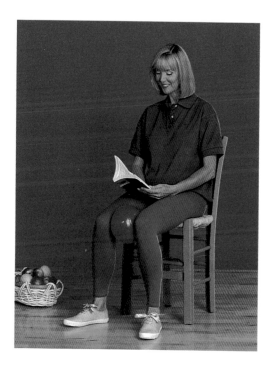

87

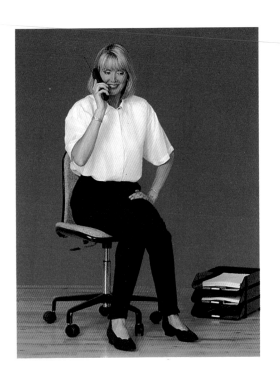

◄ Kneecap Kiss

This is an easy but effective exercise, perfect for when you are sitting in a compact space like a train or plane, or when you are on the telephone. Make sure the chair you sit on is not too high; you should be able to sit with your feet flat on the foor. Sit up straight with your knees together and your feet slightly apart. Squeeze your knees together, feeling the contraction of your inner thighs. Simultaneously contract the muscles of your abdomen and buttocks as in the Hip Hugger (see page 85). Hold for a count of 10, then relax. Repeat at least three times.

► Suspended Animotion

Joan Crawford was reported to have been able to sit through an entire meal doing this exercise! Just sit somewhat forward in your chair so that you do not touch the back. Keep your legs together with your knees bent and your feet flat on the floor. Now raise your feet about three inches (7.5 cm) off the floor. Keep your back straight and try to relax your arms so that the muscular contraction is entirely in your buttocks and thighs. This also strengthens your abdominal muscles to give you a flatter stomach. Hold for a count of at least five; then try to work up to a count of 10. Repeat three times.

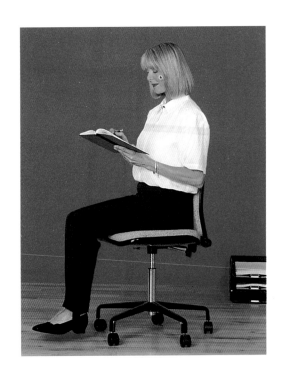

▼ **Elevator Wait Lift** *Stand with your pelvis contracted in the Hip Hugger position (see page 85), with your heels about six inches (15 cm) apart and your feet facing directly forward. Now raise your heels (**1**). You can support yourself by lightly holding on to a cabinet or the wall if necessary. Concentrate especially on the muscle tension in the hamstrings at the back of the thighs. Hold for a count of 10, then lower to the starting position. Repeat three times.*

VARIATIONS: *1. Place your heels about six inches (15 cm) apart with your toes facing diagonally out and raise your heels (**2**). Contract both your buttocks and thighs and hold for a count of 10. You will feel the muscular tension on the back sides of your thighs. Repeat three times. 2. Stand with your toes together and heels facing diagonally out, and raise your heels, for a count of 10 (**3**). Again, concentrate on the muscular contraction at the back of your thighs. Repeat three times.*

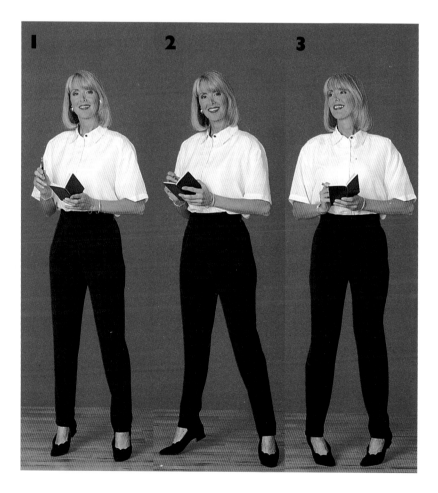

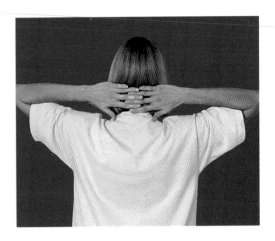

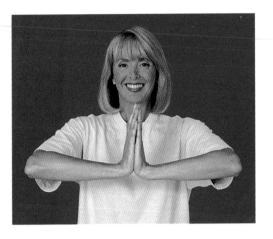

▲ **Flapper** *Intertwine your fingers behind your head, elbows bent to the side. Push your upper arms back gently as if trying to make your shoulder blades touch. Hold for 10. Repeat three times.*

▲ **Power Palm Press** *With your arms lifted in front of you at shoulder height, press your palms together for a count of 10. You will feel the tightening in your upper arms. Repeat three times.*

PRESSOMETRIC MAGIC

So, just how do Pressometrics work their magic? The answer is that isometric exercises tighten your muscles without enlarging them, automatically making you appear thinner. To prove this to yourself, just stand in front of the mirror and contract the muscles you use in the Pressometrics. Look at yourself from the front, side and back. You can see straight away that inches seem to disappear before your very eyes! You have the gratification of a "before" and "after" appearance with just one exercise.

Doing these Pressometric exercises regularly helps you to keep your muscles in a state of relative contraction so you indeed show less lumpy cellulite. You will

have concrete proof of progress within weeks, sometimes within days!

Adopt these Pressometrics as habits; the more you do, the more you will feel like doing. Start now, this minute! No matter where you are or what is going on, you can always incorporate isometric body toning into your activity. Your unconscious will soon be primed to make your daily routines into "exercise modes." At first you may need reminders. Keep a note by your toothbrush to remind you to do the Latin Lover Leg Lift first thing every morning. The cheerful ball next to your desk or telephone will remind you to do the Ball Crusher. After a while, all of these movements will become second nature. The results will be truly fantastic!

STREAMLINE STRETCHES

Before any exercise, whether it be the Twelve-Minute Miracle or aerobics, it really is important to stretch – not to warm up the muscles (since they are already warm, at body temperature) – but to ease the joints into more strenuous activity. Think of how a cat stretches as it awakens, automatically easing the transition from rest to motion.

Stretching is the basis for resculpting your body to eliminate cellulite. Elongating the muscle and the overlying lobules of fat decreases the uneven surface appearance of cellulite. The Streamline Stretches on the following pages not only prepare you for the more vigorous Twelve-Minute Miracle, but also help resculpt your cellulite-prone areas.

In performing these Streamline Stretches as well as the Twelve-Minute Miracle, move slowly into the stretch position and hold initially for a count of 10, increasing this count each day if there is no strain. This is called "static stretching." Ideally one can improve flexibility by extending the muscles as far as comfortably possible with each stretch. But do remember that, especially in stretching, it is not true that "The more it hurts, the better it is." In stretching there is only gain if there is *no* pain. When done correctly, stretches feel really good! Enjoy your own flexibility and improve at your own rhythm.

An alternative to holding the stretch is to pulsate gently. However, avoid "ballistic stretching" – bouncing in and out of the stretched position using unrestrained propulsive momentum rather than muscular control to achieve the posture, often beyond the point of comfort. Ballistic stretching lacks control, and pain is felt too late to stop the movement. Any resultant muscular damage is a temporary setback to steady improvement. The ballistic stretcher risks being out of commission for several days.

■ Stretching Tips

1. **The stretching movements should be fluid, slow, restrained, and controlled.**
2. **Never stretch beyond the range of comfort for you. With each repetition and each day you will steadily and easily increase your degree of stretch.**
3. **Concentrate. Think about each muscle as you stretch it.**
4. **Exercise initially in front of the mirror until you are quite sure of your alignment.**
5. **Hold each stretch for a count of 10. Increase the count each day if you are comfortable with the stretch.**
6. **Repeat each of the stretches at least three times. Since the Superhero Lunge is such an effective exercise for your outer and inner thighs, each type of lunge should be repeated five times on each side, followed by a second set to each side.**
7. **For extra benefit, also do the stretches *after* the Twelve-Minute Miracle.**

▶ Flamingo Stretch

1. Stand on your right foot and contract your pelvis in the Hip Hugger. Bend your left knee back, holding your pointed left foot with your left hand. Keep your knee straight down and your back straight.

2. Stretch your right arm straight up, concentrating on the stretch of the front of the left thigh and the right upper arm. Hold for a count of 10. As you improve, your arm, body, and left thigh will form a straight vertical line.

3. Now flex the left foot. Hold the position for a count of 10.

4. Repeat standing on the left foot. Repeat: three left, three right.

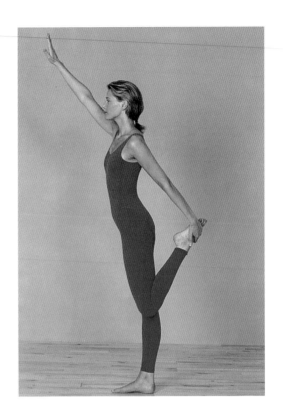

◀ Sir Walter Raleigh

1. Step forward 12–14 inches (30–36 cm) with your left heel, keeping your left leg straight with your ankle flexed and bending your right knee.

2. With your back and neck straight and your pelvis tucked in the Hip Hugger, bend your hips 90 degrees, pressing your left heel into the floor.

3. Press your hands onto your knees, feeling the stretch of both your left leg and your lifted torso. Hold for a count of 10.

4. Repeat with your right foot forward. Repeat: three left, three right.

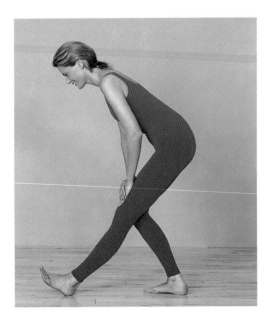

92

▶ Superhero Lunge

1. *Stand with back and neck straight, with your pelvis in the Hip Hugger position.*
2. *Step forward about 2 ½ ft (76 cm) with your left leg, turning your right foot out, and keeping your right leg straight so that your feet form a 90-degree angle (**1**).*
3. *Transfer your weight forward onto the left leg. With your heel pressed down, your left knee should be directly above, never in front of, your ankle. As you improve, your left thigh will be lower, parallel to the floor. You will feel the contraction on the outer thigh (the quadricep) of the forward (left) leg and the stretch on the inner thigh (the adductor) of the straightened (right) leg. Hold for a count of 10.*

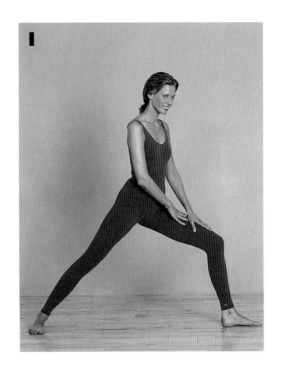

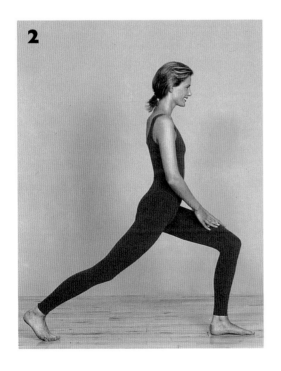

4. *Keeping the same stance, relax, turn your right foot so that it faces forward. Keeping your leg straight and lifting your right heel off the floor, stretch the right quadriceps (**2**). Hold for a count of 10.*
5. *The greater the distance between your feet, the better the stretch on your back, (straight) leg. Increase the length of stance as much as you can each day without strain. Keep your back straight at all times; do not lean forward.*
Repeat: five left, five right.
VARIATIONS: *1. Pulsate gently 10 times. 2. Place the forward foot on an elevated support such as a chair or stair.*

93

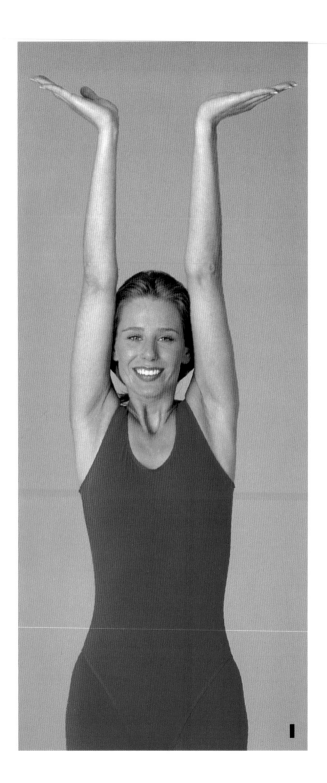

▶ Atlas Arm Stretch

*1. Lift your arms straight above your head, with palms up and fingers out (**1**). Pretend you are holding the world in your hands for a count of 10.*

2. Turn your wrists out; touch your fingertips together and stretch upward for a count of 10.

3. Repeat this stretch first with wrists in, then out, each for a count of 10 as follows:

*a: Arms straight out in front (**2**).*

*b: Arms down at sides (**3**).*

4. Repeat the stretch first with palms up and wrists straight, then with palms down and wrists flexed, each for a count of 10 as follows:

*a: Arms straight out to sides (**4**),(**5**).*

*b: Arms straight out behind you as if you were trying to make your shoulder blades, and thumbs or little fingers, respectively, touch (**6**).*

Repeat: three times.

VARIATIONS: *1. Pulsate very gently 10 times with each stretch.*

2. If you feel comfortable, wear 1 to 4lb (½ to 2kg) weights on each wrist.

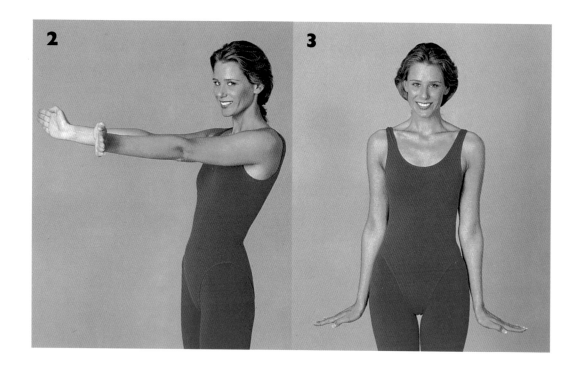

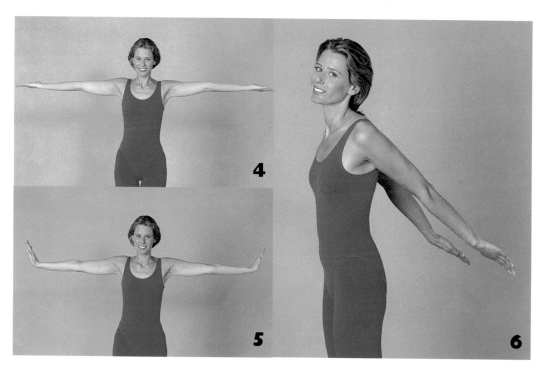

TWELVE-MINUTE MIRACLE

This exercise routine was developed partially following the ancient therapeutic art of Hatha yoga, which teaches improvement of posture and muscle tone through stretching techniques. In focusing on the muscles and correct breathing, yoga enhances concentration and increases energy. The Twelve-Minute Miracle exercises are based as well on ballet movements, which also stretch and tone.

Why yoga and ballet? Because ballet dancers and women who practice yoga have no cellulite! The fat responsible for the dimpled appearance of cellulite is just under the skin and over the muscle. Body building exercises increase muscle mass, increasing the pressure on the connective tissue packages of fat so the rippled appearance of cellulite becomes more apparent. Exercises that stretch the muscles and tendons also stretch the overlying fat layer, so that the uneven, mattress-like appearance disappears.

Do not be intimidated by feeling that you do not have the flexibility or balance to even attempt such lofty arts as yoga or ballet. These movements are simple and graceful. You can work at your own pace. You need not push your limits; this is not a contest; you don't need grit-your-teeth discipline. There *is* gain without pain! These exercises are peaceful and relaxing. You will be invigorated and happy after your sessions and proud that you accomplished some improvement each day.

■ Exercise Tips

1. It is vital to *develop the habit* of doing the Twelve-Minute Miracle exercises regularly once or twice each day. No matter how busy you are, you can always set aside twelve minutes – especially when you see how much they improve you!

2. As you do each movement – whether it be a stretch, an isometric contraction, an exercise routine, an aerobic, or a sport – *focus on form.* Think about the muscles used in each movement. When you do the exercise routine, move steadily, with control; do not fling yourself into each position using momentum, use controlled muscular contraction.

3. Never strain. Listen to your body and work at your own pace. Do not think of exercise as a personal contest; you need not push yourself; just attempt to do today at least what you did yesterday. You can start doing each repetition three times; when you are comfortable with that, increase to five, then seven, then 10. Then begin to hold the postures for a bit longer, concentrating on your muscular contractions. It is even good from time to time to touch your contracted muscle to feel how effectively you are exercising.

4. Never hold your breath as you exercise! You should inhale in the passive movement and exhale with the active movement. Let deep breathing relax you; think of the oxygen which is carrying energy to your stretched or contracted muscles with each breath you take.

Twelve-minute miracle at a glance

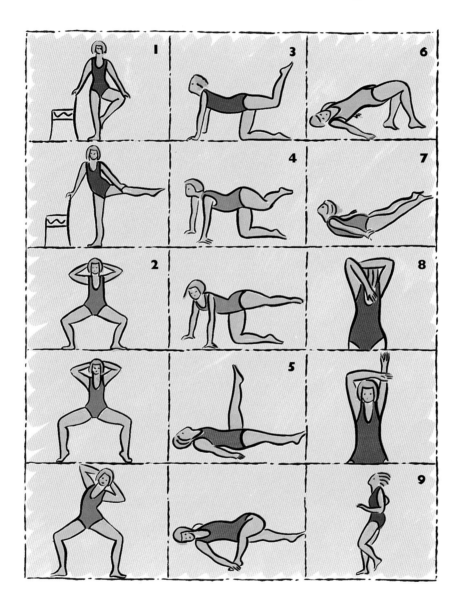

1 *Kick 'em Out*	4 *Thigh High Side Stretch*	7 *Floor Glider*
2 *Low-High Spring*	5 *Metronome*	8 *Semaphore Wave*
3 *Thigh High Back Kick*	6 *Bungee Buns*	9 *Happy Hundred*

▶ Kick 'em Out

1. Stand with your heels together and your toes turned comfortably outwards. With your right hand, hold lightly on to a waist-high support, such as a bureau or the back of a steady chair.

2. With your toe pointed and your knee out to the side, bend your left leg until your toe touches the inner side of your right knee (1). Keep your back straight and tighten your buttocks in the Hip Hugger position, pushing your left knee back as far as you can do so comfortably. As you practice, you will be able to increase your "turn out." Do not strain.

3. Extend your left leg straight out to the side without moving your hips (2).

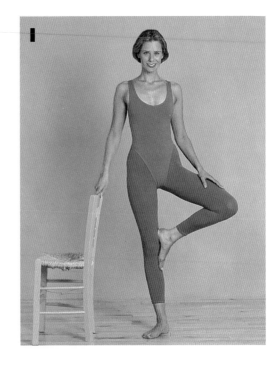

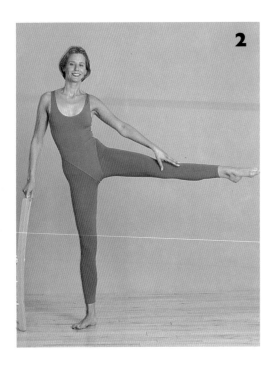

Slightly turn your pointed foot so that your heel faces the wall directly in front of you. Hold this position for a count of five.

4. Flex your foot for a count of five; then point again for a count of five.

5. Bring your extended leg in again to the position in Step 2 and lift your bent (left) knee up slightly for a count of five before returning to the starting position.

Repeat: five left, five right.

VARIATIONS: *1. After turning your heel toward the wall in front of you, turn it toward the wall behind you and hold for a count of five, first with the toes pointed, then flexed, then pointed again.*

2. If you feel comfortable wear 1 to 4lb (½ to 2kg) ankle weights. Do not strain.

▼ Low-High Spring

1. *Stand with your feet a little more than shoulder-width apart, knees bent and toes turned diagonally out. Keep your hands behind your head with your elbows pointing outwards.*

2. *Bend your knees so that your thighs are as close to horizontal as is comfortable for you, keeping your heels on the ground and your buttocks tightened in the Hip Hugger position (**1**). Hold for a count of five.*

Never allow your buttocks to drop below the level of your knees.

3. *Relax and then rise to your toes for a count of five, keeping buttocks and thighs tight in the Hip Hugger position (**2**).*

4. *Return to the starting position. Bend sideways from the waist; towards your left knee (**3**). Hold for a count of five. Then straighten and bend to the right, towards the right knee; hold for a count of five. Repeat: five times.*

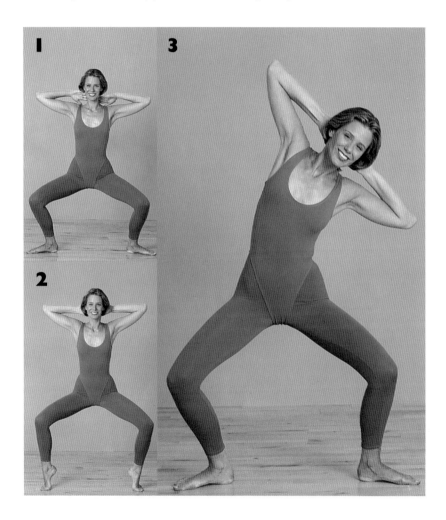

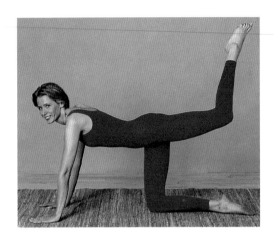

▲ Thigh High Back Kick

1. Kneel on the floor with your knees apart, positioned under your hip bones, and your elbows straight. Keep your buttocks tight in the Hip Hugger position; do not let your back or neck arch.

2. Lift your bent left leg behind you, forming a straight line from head to knee. Reach for the ceiling with your toe. The movement is very subtle. Hold the position for a count of five.

3. Flex your foot, reaching for the ceiling with your heel; hold for a count of five.

4. Repeat with pointed toe again.

Repeat: five left, five right.

▼ Thigh High Side Stretch

1. Kneel on all fours on the floor with your knees apart, positioned under your hip bones, and your arms directly under your shoulders with elbows relaxed, not locked. Keep your stomach and buttocks tight in the Hip Hugger position.

2. Keeping your knee bent, lift your left leg out to the side with your thigh parallel to the floor (**1**).

3. Without moving your hips, straighten the bent leg, keeping it out to the side and actively stretch with pointed toe (**2**).

4. Subtly twist your leg, first so that the sole of your foot reaches towards the ceiling, then slowly twist so that it reaches towards the floor. This twist is very effective in stretching your thigh muscles.

5. Repeat the stretch and twist with your foot flexed.

6. Repeat with your toes pointed.

7. Return first to Step 2, then to the starting position.

Repeat: five left, five right.

VARIATION: If you feel comfortable wear 1 to 4lb (½ to 2kg) weights on your ankles. Do not ever strain.

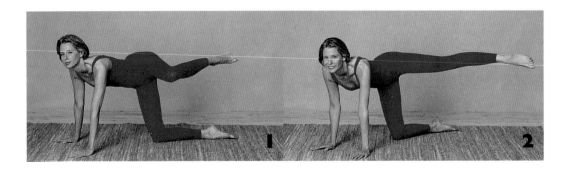

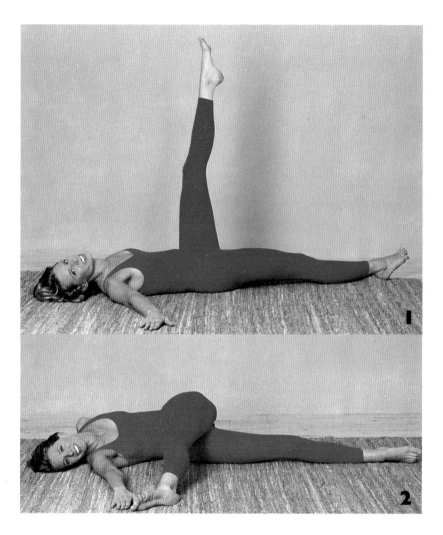

▲ Metronome

1. *Lie on the floor on your back with your arms stretched out to the sides, toes pointed, forming a T-shape.*

2. *Lift your left leg straight up, stretching your pointed toe as though you were trying to touch the ceiling (**1**).*

3. *Then flex your foot, and stretch as though you were trying to touch your heel to the ceiling.*

4. *Again, point your toe and stretch your leg upward.*

5. *Now cross your left leg over your body to touch your right hand (**2**). Tap the floor beside your hand three times with your pointed toe, then with your heel, and again with your toe.*

6. *Repeat Steps 2-4 before returning to the starting position.*

Repeat: five left, five right.

101

▼ Bungee Buns

1. Lie on your back with your knees apart and bent and your feet flat on the floor about hip distance apart. Place your palms flat on the floor with your arms at your sides, slightly away from your body for support.

2. Lift your pelvis, forming a straight line from knees to shoulders.

3. Now tuck into the Hip Hugger position, subtly raising your pelvis. Hold for a count of 10; release. Repeat five times.

4. In the contracted Hip Hugger position, bring your knees together, holding for a count of 10. You will feel the contractions in your inner thighs.

Repeat: five times.

▼ Floor Glider

1. Lie face down, with straight legs (either together or apart) and arms stretched straight out at the sides, palms down.

2. Raise your chest and arms as high as possible. You should be looking straight ahead. Think of yourself doing a swan dive, or gliding like a svelte seagull. Hold for a count of five.

3. Lower your chest and arms and raise both legs as high as possible. Hold for a count of five.

4. A variation (see photograph) is to raise your chest, arms and legs simultaneously and hold for a count of five. Do this only when and if it is comfortable for you.

Repeat: three times.

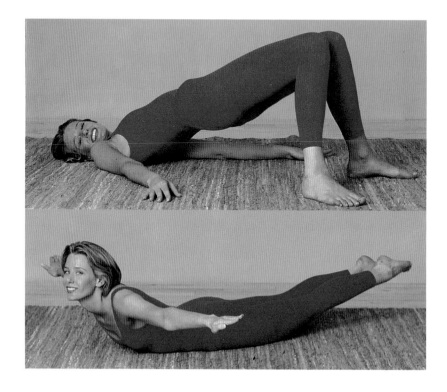

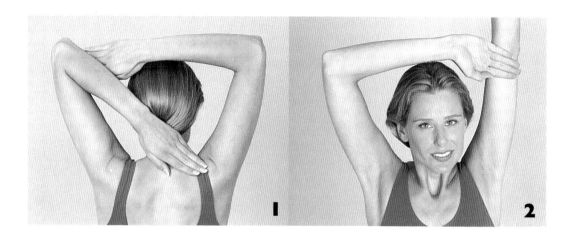

▲ Semaphore Wave

1. Standing straight with your pelvis tucked in the Hip Hugger position, raise your left arm straight up and bend your elbow so that your palm touches your left shoulder blade. Press your right hand with palm forward against your left elbow, pushing your elbow back for a count of 10 (**1**). You will feel the stretch in the triceps.
2. Extend your left arm straight above your head, turning your palm back (**2**). Stretch upward for a count of 10 and return to the starting position.
Repeat: five times.

▶ Happy Hundred

Wearing supportive running shoes, run in place for 100 steps, lifting your knees high and swinging your arms. Land on the balls of your feet with bent knees, allowing your heels to touch the floor. For variety, do jumping jacks or can-can kicks, skip or jump rope.

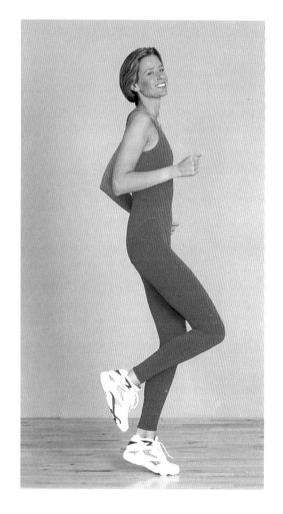

AEROBIC EXERCISE

Think of how children move: they run with their whole bodies, moving their arms actively. They dash about, climbing whenever possible, running instead of walking, while adults move slowly and deliberately. Our society discourages movement: we sit in offices, in cars, in front of TVs. We take elevators instead of climbing stairs; we ride, even short distances, rather than walk.

You can increase your aerobic exercise easily every day without setting aside any special exercise time by following two simple rules:

1. Never ride when instead you could walk or climb. I am not suggesting anything unreasonable. If it takes more than 20-30 minutes to walk to work, walking might be quite inconvenient. If your office is on the 103rd floor of the New York Trade Tower, the two-hour climb would be a bit much. However, you could always get off the bus one stop early or walk the last few flights of stairs. Walk to work in exercise shoes and keep your "professional" shoes at the office.

2. Whenever you walk or climb stairs, make an effort to move a little bit faster than your natural pace. Burn a few more calories with a little more action!

These seemingly small increases in exercise really add up, especially if you increase your activity incrementally each day. If your weight is 140 pounds (10 st/64 kg), by walking 10 minutes extra each day and climbing only four flights of stairs, you burn at least 17,500 calories each year. You could lose 5 pounds (2.3 kg) instead of gaining an average of 1 pound (0.4 kg) from inactivity.

Although the special Twelve-Minute Miracle exercises do reshape your body if you do them regularly, and dieting does help you lose extra fat, for permanent body fat loss, aerobic exercise really is necessary. And the results are immediate!

To understand just how essential aerobic exercise is for losing weight, it is important to learn how the body generates energy. The word "aerobic" means that the muscles "use oxygen" as their energy source. Aerobic exercise does not require that a person be out of breath or exhausted – in fact, quite the contrary – but it must be of long enough duration to have the desired effect.

In aerobic exercise, the body gets extra oxygen by the heart's beating faster, pumping more blood through the lungs, increasing the uptake of oxygen and transporting it to muscles to burn calories. Any exercise, therefore, can be aerobic if it is sustained for more than a short time, causing the pulse rate to increase. In contrast, intense exercises which require short spurts of energy – such as a 50-yd (46 m) dash or weight-lifting or any fast-moving sports such as squash – are anaerobic (the word means "without oxygen"). In the first burst of any movement, the activated muscles burn their stored phosphates for fuel. For the next few minutes of the exercise, energy is generated from the conversion of glycogen, stored in the muscles and liver, to glucose, a process called glycolysis. Glycolysis generates lactic acid, the waste product responsible for "the burn" in exercise. As soon as any exercise begins, there is increased uptake of oxygen. However, it takes a few minutes before aerobic metabolism generates energy. By the time the glycogen is depleted, energy begins to be generated by the aerobic burning of fat.

Although there is naturally some use of muscle and liver glycogen in all exercise, 99 percent of the energy in steady exercise is aerobic. Aerobic exercise uses stored fat from all over the body (subcutaneous fat as well as the fat cushioning organs and the tiny strands of fat between muscle fibers) as fuel, just as a fire uses oxygen to burn coal or wood.

Fat is a dense fuel: while glucose only contains 4 calories of energy per gram, fat contains 9 calories per gram. That's why fatty foods are fattening! Though they give more calories of energy, if that energy is not used, it is stored as fat.

The benefits of aerobic exercise to health are very, very important:

1. *Fat is burned.* Aerobic exercise is the most effective way to lose fat. It is a myth, however, that fat turns to muscle. (Unused muscle withers and is replaced by fat.) Aerobic exercise burns fat as it maintains and builds muscle.

2. *Cardiovascular fitness is increased in two ways.* First, the heart muscle becomes stronger so that it pumps more blood with each stroke. With this increased efficiency, the heart beats more slowly when you are inactive, but with exercise, the increased heart rate gives an even greater increase in oxygenation with each stroke, so you can exercise more intensely and for longer. Second, there is a significant decrease in coronary artery disease in those individuals who exercise.

3. *Aerobic exercise helps the skeletal system.* Joints become more flexible with a fuller range of motion, and the bones are strengthened by improved bone remodeling. Even in post-menopausal women, exercise has been shown to increase bone mineral content.

4. *Exercise may decrease the risk of certain kinds of cancer.* There is evidence to suggest that even moderate aerobic exercise (such as walking only two miles (3.2 km) in 30-40 minutes each day, six days per week) decreases not only the overall death rate and the number of deaths due to heart disease, but also the number of deaths due to cancer. Other research suggests that regular strenuous exercise lowers the risk of cancer of the breast and reproductive system.

5. *Aerobic exercise raises the basal metabolic rate (BMR).* This means that the body burns more calories for every activity, even resting. This is in contrast to dieting, which decreases the BMR: when

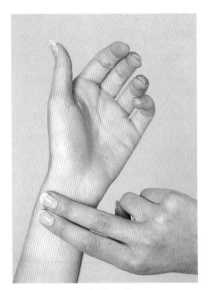

Radial pulse

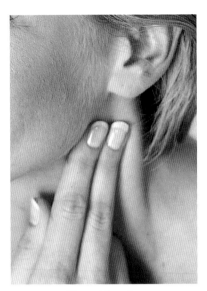

Carotid pulse

given less food, the body conserves its use of energy in preparation for famine. On the other hand, exercise maintains and builds muscle, thereby maintaining or increasing the BMR. Muscle is 37.5 times more active metabolically than the same weight of fat. One pound (0.4 kg) of fat requires only 2 calories per day, whereas one pound (0.4 kg) of muscle requires 75 calories per day. Aerobic exercise really does change body composition so that fat is reduced and muscle is increased.

There has been a controversy in medical literature as to whether exercise actually increases the metabolic rate for hours immediately after the exercise. The theory that it does was based on a frequently cited study done by a Harvard professor in the 1930s. The metabolic rates of football players were measured before and after

Use your second and third fingers to check your pulse rate either on your wrist (radial pulse) or at your neck (carotid pulse). Count the beats for 15 seconds and multiply by 4 to get the number of beats per minute.

their game, showing increased metabolic rates for 48 hours after the game.

Although recent very careful monitoring of volunteers after exercising did show that exercising very intensely for long times does indeed increase metabolism for up to three days after the exercise, moderate exercise (such as jogging for one-half hour or an aerobic calisthenics with only 20 minutes of rigorous exercise) did not give a substantial increase in metabolism, even several hours after the exercise. This should not discourage anyone from exercising – there is still the caloric effect from the exercise itself and a short period of increased metabolism after exercise when breathing is faster to provide more oxygen than the usual resting state.

6. *Exercise decreases appetite.* Led by Jean Mayer at Harvard University, many researchers have proved that sedentary individuals actually eat more than active ones. The good news is that the more sedentary and overweight a person is, the more their appetite will decrease with movement. This effect may be partially psychological, but there is also a physiological explanation: hunger is partly caused by a drop in blood sugar levels. Since muscles use far more fat than sugar as fuel, regular exercise keeps blood sugar levels more stable. Also, with exercise there is less insulin in the blood which would otherwise lower blood sugar levels.

"If it weren't for the fact that the TV set and the refrigerator are so far apart, some of us wouldn't get any exercise at all," says the New York columnist Joey Adams. So, instead of heading for the refrigerator immediately whenever you start to feel hungry, force yourself to do just 10 or 20 minutes of aerobic movement first. Maybe you won't even want that snack! Try exercising regularly before meals to suppress your appetite.

7. *Exercise really does make the body look better.* It gives tone and definition where there might otherwise be flab! Only with exercise can you resculpt your body

to pass the most stringent test of all – the "Reflection Reaction." The true criterion of how you look is not weight, not percentage of fat, not inches, but just plain how you look. Exercise always makes you look better, even if you gain a little weight in replacing light fat with denser muscle.

8. *Exercise exhilarates.* It is a natural anti-depressant! Even mild exercise stimulates the production and release of endorphins, the body's own pleasure opiates. Trained athletes often describe feeling "high." Endorphins have been shown to control appetite and to reduce anxiety. Perhaps due to endorphin release, exercise wards off depression, often a cause of overeating. Compulsive behavior cannot be considered healthful, but exercise can be addictive in a good sense. The more you exercise, the more you *can* exercise and *want* to exercise.

The Table of Energy Output on page 111 lists the caloric expenditure of various aerobic activities over and above your sedentary daily energy output. Using this table, you can calculate your energy expenditure for the Twelve-Minute Miracle (which is relatively little) and for the aerobic exercise you choose. When you add that number to your baseline daily energy output (see chart on page 109), you can determine the total number of calories burned each day. For each additional 3,500 calories that you use, you lose 1 pound (0.4 kg) of extra weight. Keeping a diary of your activity helps you realize how "expensive' that midnight snack can be in requiring exercise to compensate for those extra calories! Just the way you balance your check book, learn to calculate your calorie "balance" daily!

The great news is that the more overweight you are, the more calories you use and the more weight you will lose exercising. Just sitting at rest, a person produces about one kilocalorie (commonly called calories) per hour for each 2.2 pounds (1 kg) of body weight. You can approximate the number of kilocalories for your daily resting energy requirement (RE) (equal to your basal metabolic rate or BMR) from the table opposite.

To estimate your baseline daily energy output, add to your BMR 300 calories if on that day you are primarily inactive, 500 calories if you are moderately active, and 700 calories if you are very active.

Baseline Daily Energy Output (calories)

$$= BMR + \begin{matrix} 300 \text{ (inactive)} \\ 500 \text{ (moderately active)} \\ 700 \text{ (very active)} \end{matrix}$$

Walking

Walking is the best exercise – especially for anyone who has not been active for a while and for busy individuals who do not have time to change clothes, warm up, shower, and redress as needed to go jogging. Anyone can go for a walk (even in office clothes) by simply changing shoes. You can walk anywhere, anytime. You do not need a treadmill or a track! You can walk outside for the fun of changing scenes and getting fresh air. You can walk in place at home while watching television or with music to set your pace. You can walk alone to meditate or you can walk at a planned time with a friend.

■ Aerobic Tips

1. The optimal intensity of aerobic exercise is such that your heart rate should be 70 to 85 percent of your own maximal heart rate (beats per minute or bpm). This is high enough to give an effective workout, yet low enough that you can sustain it for 20 to 40 minutes.

Maximal heart rate (bpm) = 220 - age (yrs)

Optimal exercise heart rate (bpm) = (0.70 to 0.85) x maximal heart rate

2. Never push yourself too quickly! Even if you do not achieve 70 percent of your maximal heart rate at first, just do the exercise continuously at your own pace for at least 20 minutes. If you want you can increase the pace and duration slightly each day.
3. Exercise to music you enjoy in order to prevent boredom. Increasing the tempo week by week motivates you to increase the pace without strain.
4. Choose an aerobic activity that is convenient and fun!

■ Daily Resting Energy Requirements

Weight *(Woman aged 30)*

Pounds	90	100	110	120	130	140	150	160	170	180
Stone	6.4	7.1	7.9	8.6	9.3	10.0	10.7	11.4	12.1	12.9
Kilograms	40.8	45.4	49.9	54.4	59.0	63.5	68.0	72.6	77.1	81.6

Height (ft.) **Calories**

Height (ft.)										
4'9"	1173	1216	1260	1303	1346	1390	1433	1476	1520	1563
4'10"	1178	1221	1264	1308	1351	1394	1438	1481	1524	1568
4'11"	1182	1226	1269	1312	1356	1399	1442	1486	1529	1572
5'0"	1187	1230	1274	1317	1360	1404	1447	1490	1534	1577
5'1"	1192	1235	1278	1322	1365	1408	1452	1495	1539	1582
5'2"	1196	1240	1283	1326	1370	1413	1457	1500	1543	1587
5'3"	1201	1244	1288	1331	1374	1418	1461	1505	1548	1591
5'4"	1206	1249	1292	1336	1379	1423	1466	1509	1553	1596
5'5"	1210	1254	1297	1341	1384	1427	1471	1514	1557	1601
5'6"	1215	1258	1302	1345	1389	1432	1475	1519	1562	1605
5'7"	1220	1263	1307	1350	1393	1437	1480	1523	1567	1610
5'8"	1225	1268	1311	1355	1398	1441	1485	1528	1571	1615
5'9"	1229	1273	1316	1359	1403	1446	1489	1533	1576	1619
5'10"	1234	1277	1321	1364	1407	1451	1494	1537	1581	1624
5'11"	1239	1282	1325	1369	1412	1455	1499	1542	1586	1629
6'0"	1243	1287	1330	1373	1417	1460	1503	1547	1590	1634

These estimations of daily resting energy requirements are calculated from the Harris Benedict Equation for a woman of 30. If you are 20 years old, you should add 47 cals to the number on the chart, if you are 40 subtract 47 cals, at 50 subtract 94 cals, at 60 subtract 140 cals.

The Harris-Benedict equation for predicting resting energy requirements (RE) is

For women: $RE(cal) = 655.1 + 9.56W + 1.85H - 4.68A$

For men: $RE(cal) = 66.5 + 13.75W + 5.00H - 6.78A$

where W = weight (in kg), H = height (cm), A = age (in years)

Original reference: Harris, JA, and Benedict, FG. A biometric study of basal metabolism in man. Washington, Carnegie Institute of Washington Publ. no. 279, 1919.

■ What Are the Most Strenuous Activities?

	Inactive	Moderately Active	Very Active
Home	Driving a car Eating Hairsetting and makeup Making beds Playing music Telephone Television Waiting in line Washing dishes	Cleaning (dusting, vacuuming) Cooking Laundry, ironing Taking care of children Sexual foreplay Shopping Showering and dressing Window	Chopping wood Climbing stairs Gardening Playing with children Scrubbing floor Sexual intercourse Shovelling snow Cleaning
Work	Bank teller Driver Receptionist Secretary Student Telephone operator Typist Writer	Architect Actress Bartender Doctor Engineer Flight attendant Laboratory technician Musician Salesperson	Construction worker Dancer Farmer Mechanic Nurse Singer Teacher Waiter

For optimal benefit, (1) walk with a long stride; (2) actively swing your arms like a pendulum with each step; and (3) place the heel of your leading foot down before the toe. After you have increased your pace comfortably, you may want to add one pound (450g) wrist weights or just carry a can of soda in each hand.

Jogging

In today's hectic world, we seem to run everywhere: to work, to catch a bus or to make a meeting on time. And now many people do the "in" exercise of the decade: jogging. Recently, however, orthopedists and exercise physiologists have discovered that jogging can cause injuries to knees, legs, and backs. My advice to confirmed joggers is to jog only where there is fresh air (not in the pollution of traffic or industry), to wear good supportive shoes, to jog on a soft surface (not concrete), and to be moderate, not compulsive or excessive. I recommend fast walking instead of jogging since there is less danger of injury due to impact and

■ Energy Output Extra Calories

Weight	lbs	120	140	160	180
	kg	54.5	63.6	72.7	81.8
	stone	8.6	10.0	11.4	12.9
The Twelve Minute Miracle		75	110	130	142
Isometrics		82	96	108	126
Basketball		135	160	184	204
Bicycle	<10 mph (16 km/h)	82	96	108	126
	10-12 mph (16-19 km/h)	135	160	184	204
	12-14 mph (19-23 km/h)	190	224	254	286
	14-16 mph (23-26 km/h)	246	286	330	370
Calisthenics	moderate	95	112	127	146
	vigorous	190	224	254	286
Climbing steps		190	224	254	286
Golf	using cart	68	80	90	104
	rolling clubs	118	128	142	164
Dancing (ballet, modern, twist, or disco)		135	160	184	204
Horseback riding		82	96	108	126
Jumping rope	slow	190	224	254	286
	moderate	246	286	330	370
	fast	300	350	400	450
Tennis	doubles	135	160	184	204
	singles	190	224	254	286
Rebounding		68	80	90	104
Rowing, stationary	light	68	80	90	104
	moderate	166	192	218	248
	vigorous	205	240	272	380
Running	5 mph (12 min/mile) (8 km/h)	190	224	254	286
	6 mph (10 min/mile) (10 km/h)	246	286	330	370
	7 mph (8 min/mile) (11 km/h)	310	355	418	470
Swimming (freestyle, backstroke) moderate		190	224	254	286
	fast	246	286	330	370
Tai Chi		82	96	108	126
Walking	2 mph (3 km/h)	40	48	55	62
	3 mph (5 km/h)	68	80	90	104
	4 mph (6 km/h)	82	96	108	126
Yoga		82	96	108	126

The number of calories greater than a sedentary activity (burned during 30 minutes of each activity)

walking can burn as many calories as jogging. (Walking two miles in 30 minutes burns the same number of extra calories as jogging one mile in 10 minutes).

Skipping Rope

Skipping rope is as effective as jogging in burning calories and has the advantage that it can be done indoors or out. An old clothesline or extension cord (not plugged in!) and well padded shoes are all you need. Since even the lowest rate requires a lot of energy, jump for two to three minute intervals, walking in place in between. Music really helps. Be sure to jump on the balls of your feet and to alternate feet in a skipping action; do not jump with both feet at the same time.

Climbing Steps

Walking up stairs exercises the entire body. If you work or live on an upper floor, this is an ideal exercise. Even if you walk halfway, you gain by climbing the first few flights. Walking up stairs is far better than using an expensive, indoor step machine. You burn fewer calories on the latter since you need not pick up your feet, and you may lean on the rails. If you do not have steps in your home or in your office, just step up and down on a thick book, preferably to music. If you have bad knees, don't climb stairs for fitness.

Swimming

Swimming can be done at any age even when other activities might be limited by injury or diseased such as arthritis. Swimming uses your whole body and is impact free; there is no stress on joints.

Extra calories burned in 30 minutes of exercise if you weigh 140 lbs

Jumping rope: .286 cal
Golf: . . . . .128 cal
Rebounding: . . . . .80 cal
Playing ball: .160 cal
Kite flying: . . . . .100 cal
Jogging: . . . . .286 cal
Yoga: . . . . .96 cal

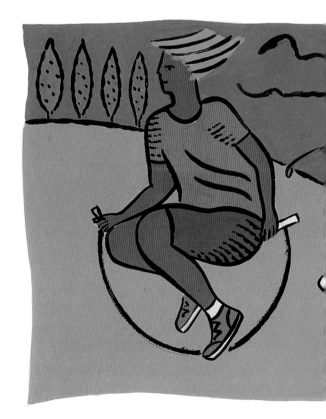

The resistance of water increases the intensity of any workout. To maximize the benefits, think about your thigh and arm muscles with each stroke, contracting your thighs as you kick. Cup your hands or hold small paddles to increase the resistance and maximize the exercise. You need not limit yourself to swimming laps. You can walk vigorously across the pool in shoulder-high water; you can do kicks and stretches while holding on to the side.

Rebounding

A rebounder is a springy mat like a miniature trampoline except that the fabric and construction are designed for only a little spring, not to catapult acrobats into the air. The rebounder (which is inexpensive) allows you to do all aerobic jumping (jogging, jumping jacks, hopping, kicking) without the danger of impact injuries. The calories burned depend upon the activity. Rebounding exercise is an especially good way for a sedentary person to begin exercising. It is even possible for an elderly person or an invalid to benefit by bouncing the hips in a sitting position or to exercise the legs alone with someone else jumping. People with difficulty in balance should not use a rebounder.

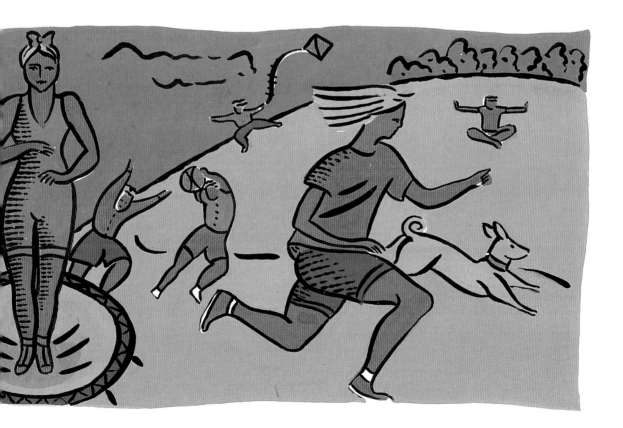

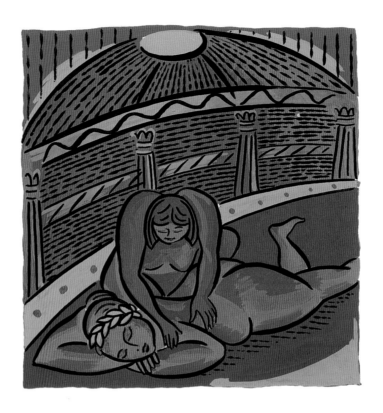

Massage: from the skin in

As a dermatologist with a lifetime of research in slowing the ageing of the skin, I daily observe the skin as an important and fascinating metabolic organ. Far more than just our outer wrapping, it is our protection from injury, from radiation, and from infectious agents. The skin has an immune system which helps to regulate fluid balance, produces vitamin D, regulates body temperature by both shivering or sweating, and makes its own moisturizer – by far the most effective skin "conditioner" that exists!

What does the skin have to do with cellulite? Although, as you learned in Chapter 2, the condition of cellulite originates *under* the skin, its unattractive appearance, as we are all well aware is very much on the surface!

There are easy strategies to make your skin look its best. Skin brushing and massage have been a part of skin care for sensual luxury, for beautification, and for health for many centuries. Skin brushing rids your skin of dead cells and gives it a polished, youthful smoothness. And massage stimulates circulation and lymphatic drainage, improving exchange between blood, lymph and fat cells and connective tissue – all beneficial effects.

In this chapter you will learn special techniques that definitely help to reduce the lumpy appearance of cellulite. You need spend only five minutes each day to see an improvement and to help keep your body cellulite-free. Be aware, though, that these methods are not a substitute for maintaining your proper weight and toning your muscles. If all you're willing to do is lie on a massage table, don't expect any progress! In combination with your GREFLOF Eating Plan, your Pressometrics and your Twelve-Minute Miracle, however, these skin care routines do complement your improvement and help to preserve your well-earned cellulite-free body.

Your Enemy the Sun

To have your skin look its best, your single most important act is to *protect yourself from the sun*. None of us is immune to the very dangerous effects of the sun; people with lighter skin are at added risk. Although tanned skin may appear to act as camouflage for the dimples of cellulite, *all* sun exposure is bad. There is no such thing as a safe tan!

The sun prematurely ages your skin. Just compare the skin at the top of your inner arm with the skin on the back of your hand. Anyone over 30 will notice that the non-sun-exposed skin of the inner arm is supple and smooth, quite different from that of the more wrinkled sun-exposed hand. With extreme sun exposure, the skin becomes leathery, with loss of elasticity and blotchy dark and sometimes rough spots (which may be precancerous).

The sun causes skin cancer, especially in those individuals with moles, with a previous skin cancer or a family history of skin cancer. Ever since designer Coco Chanel shocked the fashion world of the 1920s by showing her Paris couture collection on tanned models, successive generations have accepted tanned skin as one of the hallmarks of an exclusive, healthy lifestyle. Today's medical evidence is very clearly to the contrary. *Tanning is actually the visible evidence of damage to your skin* – the very same damage that causes premature wrinkling, dark spots and skin cancer.

You should *not* sit and bake in the sun - ever! Stay out of the sun during the peak hours of 10am to 3pm. If you are fair-skinned and live in a northern climate be especially cautious when vacationing in sunny places. Going south in the winter or skiing (with the strong reflection of the sun off the snow) can give you severe sunburn. Outdoors, use a waterproof sunscreen of sun protection factor (SPF) 25 to 30 all year round. Apply sunscreen about 20 minutes before going out, and reapply every two hours when swimming or perspiring from exercise.

Don't ever go to a tanning salon! Although they may promise a "safe" tan from "blacklight" with only lower energy UVA radiation (sunlight is UVA + UVB), forget it! Unlike UVB, UVA does not directly cause skin cancer, but it does damage the deeper layers of skin, causing irreversible ageing by destroying structural proteins and harming the skin's immune system, decreasing its ability to fight infection. If you really think that you look better tanned, especially on the areas where you have cellulite, use a self-tanning cream. If you incorporate a few minutes of skin brushing into your daily beauty routine, you'll need to re-apply self-tanner daily since you will have removed the outer layer of skin with each brushing. "Tan from a bottle" does look good if evenly applied, but beware: it gives no protection from the sun. So-called tanning accelerators containing psoralin to activate

UVA-induced tanning are actually dangerous. They should be avoided unless prescribed by a physician for the medical treatment of a disease.

SKIN BRUSHING

In Japan, Sweden, and other countries, dry skin brushing is a part of a woman's daily hygiene. In Europe it is increasingly popular. Dry brushing removes the dead cells that stick to the outer layer of skin, actually "sanding" and "polishing" the skin to a youthful luster and a silky smooth texture. Dry brushing not only enhances the appearance and texture of the skin, but also acts physiologically in two ways that directly reduce cellulite:
1. There is increased turnover of skin cells and connective tissue. The surface skin is renewed and the collagen septae are remodelled more rapidly.
2. There is increased blood flow within the vast network of capillaries in the deep layer of skin and in the subcutaneous fat, as well as improvement of lymphatic flow.

Although many types of anti-cellulite "body smoothers" are sold, for truly effective dry skin brushing I recommend a massage glove with stiff, densely spaced natural bristles. Brush your entire body. You may find it more comfortable to stand, with the leg you are brushing lifted onto a stool or a chair. The direction of brushing should always be from the extremities to the top of the leg or arm, following the return blood flow to the heart. Start with your feet, then brush your legs and calves, thighs, buttocks, back stomach, and arms (from the hands to the shoulders). Brush with long sweeps on the legs and arms, and with rounded, half-circle motions on the thighs, abdomen, and back, with movements always towards the heart.

Concentrate on the sites of your worst cellulite. Brush your entire inner and outer thighs and buttocks especially vigorously several times. Don't forget the more difficult-to-reach areas just above your knees and just below your buttocks. Perhaps you'll find it easier to brush in front of a mirror to be sure you do not miss important spots. Brushing should be firm so that you feel invigorated, but do not brush too strongly – you should end with a pink glow, not with irritated, red skin. Avoid brushing any areas with rashes, cuts or inflammations.

You can also achieve some of the advantages of skin brushing by using exfoliants especially designed to remove the thick layers of dead surface skin cells. After extensive research, I have formulated for my exclusive line of Longévité® skin care products a very different exfoliant that gently adheres to dead surface cells, peeling them off. This exfoliant can also be used safely on the face to reduce the appearances of small wrinkles and enlarged pores. Other good exfoliants are those with little sandy grains. Although these must be used with caution on the

face (the particles can get into your eyes), these exfoliants are fine for the cellulitic areas of your thighs, back, and upper arms. Use the same skin brushing motions for exfoliating your body.

I recommend that you brush or exfoliate twice a day – in the morning and just before bed. Do it before your bath or shower to ensure that you are brushing or exfoliating dry skin. The entire procedure should take less than five minutes, but even one or two minutes concentrating on your areas of cellulite make a difference!

SELF-MASSAGE

Massage is one of the most relaxing and enjoyable treatments for cellulite. Massage motions actually manipulate the subcutaneous fat tissue so that circulation of blood and lymph is improved, even more than with skin brushing. Remember that increased circulation mitigates the adverse effect of blocking valves within tiny blood vessels, devices that would otherwise constrict blood flow and aggravate cellulite. However, even with these benefits, massage does not and will not dissolve fat! Massage is of little value in eliminating cellulite unless it is combined with weight loss (where appropriate) and toning through exercise.

Many beauty salons and so-called health clinics specialize in cellulite massage, often combined with special lotions or oils (which may be effective) and with body wrapping (which in fact gives only transient improvement). These expensive professional treatments offer nothing that you cannot do for yourself at home. In fact if you follow the advice in this book, you too can enjoy the advantages of the most exclusive spa! As with skin brushing, you may prefer to massage in front of a mirror to be sure that you treat completely all areas with cellulite. Always massage towards the heart. The massage should be firm, but not so traumatic that it causes bruising. I recommend that you massage twice daily, just after skin brushing.

Before you massage any area, apply a lotion, gel or oil of your choice to help your hands glide over your skin. Many new and expensive toning and anti-cellulite gels and lotions promise "complex action to slim, firm, and tighten" for "sensational body contouring". There is great controversy as to whether these products are any more effective than massaging with far less expensive lotions. Although some of these so-called anti-cellulite products contain esoteric ingredients from plants and algae (of possible but questionable efficacy), others do have components, proven effective on isolated fat cells. These scientifically studied ingredients are, believe it or not, caffeine and the structurally similar molecules theophyllin and aminophyllin. When caffeine is added to fat cells in laboratory tests, it acts on specific enzymes to inhibit transport of fat into fat cells and to break down the fat within fat cells. (One

application is equivalent to drinking less than half a cup of coffee.) Whether the caffeine is delivered effectively to the fat cell layer by massage has however not been proven definitively. I have researched and developed Longévité® Cellulite Treatment Lotion which contains not only caffeine, but also a high concentration of a natural vitamin which acts on connective tissue so that the septae surrounding fat cells remain thinner and the surface of the skin retains its elasticity longer. Despite the proven results on isolated fat cells, the effect of these ingredients on women's thighs is at best subtle and difficult to verify. A recently published study showed that after a daily five-week application of an aminiphylin-containing cream, treated thighs shrunk in circumference by about ½ inch (1 cm). Unfortunately these results cannot be considered conclusive, since measurements are not very accurate. With the known effectiveness of drugs delivered into the skin using patches, it is logical that a cream applied to the thighs can also be delivered effectively. In addition, massage heats the skin, increasing absorption. But the jury is still out, so I recommend that you try for yourself.

Although in no way a substitute for good eating and good exercise, techniques such as skin brushing and massage, combined with the right kind of lotion, can be of considerable help. You can, indeed, treat your cellulite "from the skin in." Try it! You'll relax, and feel great!

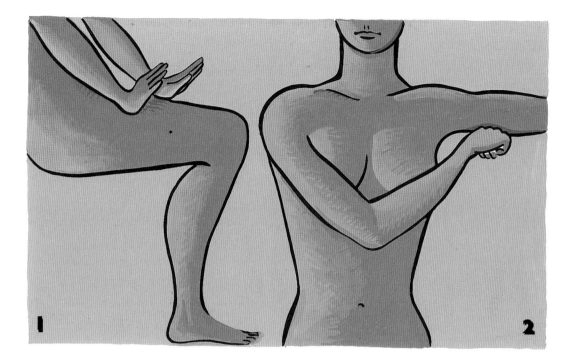

When you massage, first apply lotion, gel, or oil with a sweeping motion, applying pressure as you stroke towards the heart. Use one of three techniques:

1. The Hand Heel Technique (**1**) is best for your thighs. Bend your wrist back, lifting your palm and fingers, and firmly massage your thigh just above the knee, massaging upwards to your upper thigh. Next massage the front and back of your thigh, starting again at the knee and moving upwards. Don't forget just under your buttocks. Massage each thigh for at least one minute.

2. The Knuckle Technique (**2**) is best for your upper arms. Extend the arm to be massaged in front of you with elbow bent and make a fist with your other hand. Press your knuckles firmly along your upper arm, massaging with long strokes from the elbow to the top of the arm. Do at least 20 full strokes on each arm.

3. Although both the Hand Heel and the Knuckle Techniques are also effective for the "love handles" of the lower back, you might prefer the kneading technique called petrissage. This method can also be used on your upper arms, but do not use it for your thighs since it may encourage the formation of tiny spider veins. Grasp the fold of skin on your lower back between your thumb and fingers, squeeze and twist as if you were kneading dough. You can simultaneously massage both sides of your back for at least one minute by whichever of the three techniques you prefer.

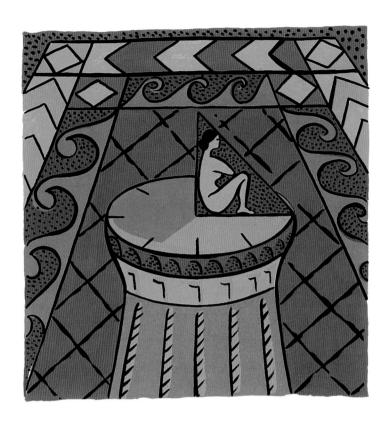

Your cellulite reduction diary

I am proud of you! You've read the entire book! You've learned the science of cellulite, so you realize that cellulite is here to stay - but you also know that the bulging, dimply appearance of your cellulite-prone areas can be improved. You can easily follow the *Simple Steps to Thin Thighs* method on your own, doing some part of your daily routine with a companion. For instance, you might enjoy exercising

YOUR CELLULITE REDUCTION DIARY

with a friend several times each week, and encouraging each other to follow the diet rules by meeting for lunch or dinner.

Either way, I find it helpful to keep a diary to "score" myself. A diary inspires me to keep going. Since my plan is carried out at home, without the advantage (or expense) of a rigidly scheduled spa or the supervision of a trainer, the discipline is entirely individual. Keeping a diary shows what you're really doing each day. Don't fall into the trap of thinking that if you read a self-improvement book, that is enough! By taking a few minutes to think about yourself, and write your thoughts down, you will identify your weak points so that you can improve. You will realize how much you have accomplished.

Even if keeping a diary is not your usual custom, I would encourage you to complete the first few lines of the diary each day. Photocopy the diary on page 123 as many times as you need. The first entry is why you are happy with yourself. Optimism and happiness help everyone. Each day actively consider one special reason to be happy: maybe today your hair or make-up really look good, or that you really did your set of the Twelve-Minute Miracle before your children awakened or your phone interrupted. Then think of an improvement to emphasize that day; by repeating to yourself a positive phrase, a sort of "Improvement Mantra," you will reinforce that behavior. "Stand tall." "Feel energy." "Breathe

deep." "Walk tight." "Squeeze that fat." "Savor each bite." By emphasizing one small good practice each day, you will soon make it a part of your life.

In the daily diary, next list your weight that day, taken in the morning with no clothes, just after awakening and emptying your bladder. Whether you are trying to lose weight or simply maintain your weight, it does help to weigh yourself each day. If you weigh more than the day before, you need only cut down what you eat that day. Eating slightly smaller portions, especially at dinner, and no desserts usually does the trick. This daily monitoring allows you to maintain your weight so that extra pounds do not slowly accumulate to the point of disaster. If you are trying to lose weight, don't be discouraged if you hit a plateau, not measurably losing for several days. As long as you don't gain much weight, you are on the right track. Some dieters prefer to weigh themselves only once each week. Do what best helps *you*!

Your next entry in the diary is your exercise goal for that day – the number of sets of Pressometrics and the Twelve-Minute Miracle and aerobic activity you plan to do. Perhaps that day there is no time for extra exercise, or perhaps it's Sunday and you can swim and play tennis all afternoon. At the end of the day, note whether you indeed accomplished your goal. Whether you did or not, the achievement or the guilt will stimulate your positive action for the next day!

You might enjoy making a game of sticking to your cellulite reduction routine by keeping score. For each set of Pressometrics and of the Twelve-Minute Miracle and for each 15 minutes of aerobics, give yourself one Slimming Star. If you did not extra-exercise at all (not even walking a few flights of stairs instead of taking the lift), give yourself one Pudgy Point. Then honestly note whether you followed your diet plan. Reward yourself with a Slimming Star for each meal that you did keep to your diet. If not, penalize yourself with one Pudgy Point. For each binge, add another Pudgy Point.

You can then see your Success Score by adding your exercise score to your diet score. By following your plan, you can achieve a high score of +7 to +10 (depending on your exercise); the lowest possible score is -5 to -8 (depending on how much you binged). It is easy to have a positive score! And even if your score is negative on one day, you can make up for it the following day.

The Weekly Review is quite important. Writing down whether you followed your diet and exercise plan and identifying your problems in keeping to it allows you to adjust and correct the following week. And do pat yourself on the back for your accomplishments. If you completed any of this *Simple Steps to Thin Thighs* program, you can proudly record your feelings for that week and the improvements you see.

Your Reflection Reaction is important! Look closely at yourself in the mirror each week. Do you look better than you did the week before, with a smoother contour over your areas of cellulite? If so, just write "+"; if not, "-"; if the same write "0".

List your weight each week. Always keep your target in mind. If you are over 30, this may be your weight when you were in your early twenties. Be sure to choose an ideal weight within 10 percent of the normal weights listed on page 47. Remember, replacing fat with muscle can slightly increase your weight, so do not be discouraged if you exercised and are a bit heavier. Each of your measurements may decrease only slightly (if at all); but you will have decreased your overall measurements after several weeks and a seemingly small loss makes a tremendous improvement in your silhouette.

Record how many days you did not cheat on your personal diet and list your exercising. I recommend that you do one or two sets of Pressometrics and the Twelve-Minute Miracle each day and aerobic activities for a total of about 2 ½ hours each week – or about 20 minutes each day, 30 minutes five days per week, or 40 minutes four days each week. Your program need not be rigid, as long as you exercise. Documenting your Weekly Review Chart will keep you on track.

Simple Steps to Thin Thighs means for you a healthier, more enjoyable life. You'll feel better, look better, and you'll have fun!

■ Daily Diary

Week number: _____ Day: _____ Date: _____ Weight: _____

Why I am happy with myself today: _____

_____

My Improvement Mantra today: _____

_____

SUCCESS SCORE

EXERCISE

		Today's goal	Today's achievement	Slimming Stars	Pudgy Points
Pressometrics	# sets	_____	_____	_____	_____
Twelve-Minute Miracle	# sets	_____	_____	_____	_____
Aerobics	time	_____	_____	_____	_____
I did no extra exercise today					_____

Exercise Score: Slimming Stars – Pudgy Points = _____

DIET

	Slimming Stars	Pudgy Points
Did I follow my diet plan today at breakfast?	_____	_____
lunch?	_____	_____
dinner?	_____	_____
snacks?	_____	_____
Did I binge today? *(each binge = 1 Pudgy Point)*		_____

Diet Score: Slimming Stars – Pudgy Points = _____

Success Score = Exercise Score + Diet Score = _____

123

■ Weekly Review Chart

	START	WK.1	WK.2	WK.3	WK.4	WK.5
Date						
Weight						
Reflection Reaction**						
Measurements (inches or cm)						
Waist						
Hip						
Upper Thigh R / L						
Mid Thigh R / L						
Low Thigh R / L						
Sum of all measurements						
Diet						
# days goal met						
Exercise						
Total # sets						
Pressometrics						
Twelve-Minute Miracle						
Aerobic hours						
Review						
Did I follow my GREFLOF plan this week?	yes / no	yes / no	yes / no	yes / no	yes / no	yes / no
Of what am I most proud in keeping on my GREFLOF plan?						
What was my biggest problem in keeping on my GREFLOF plan?						
Did I follow my exercise plan this week?	yes / no	yes / no	yes / no	yes / no	yes / no	yes / no
What was my greatest joy in exercising?						
What was my biggest problem in exercising?						
My best feeling this week:						
My best improvement this week:						
My behavior to emphasize next week:						
Success Score*						

* Total Slimming Stars minus Pudgy Points
** Grade the dimply appearance of your cellulite:
"+" if improved, "0" if the same, "-" if worse.

124

WK.6	WK.7	WK.8	WK.9	WK.10	WK.11	WK.12	GOAL
yes / no	yes / no	yes / no	yes / no	yes / no	yes / no	yes / no	yes / no
yes / no	yes / no	yes / no	yes / no	yes / no	yes / no	yes / no	yes / no

Index

adipocytes, 20
aerobics, 65, 81, 104-13
ageing, 27
alcohol, 54, 66
amino acids, 62-3
aminophyllin, 22, 118
angel food cake, 78
anorexia nervosa, 44
antioxidants, 65
appetite, exercise and, 107
apple bran muffins, 71
apple shape, 21
artichokes with garlic, 76
Atlas Arm Stretch, 94, *94-5*

baby fat, 26
Ball Crusher, 87, *87*
ballistic stretching, 91
basal metabolic rate, 105-6
basketball, 111
beauty, perception of, 8-13
bicycling, 111
bioelectric impedance, 44
blood vessels, 21, 25-6, 29, 30-1,
  116-17
bones, exercise and, 105
breakfast, 64, 68, 71
brown fat, 26
bulimia, 44
Bungee Buns, 102, *102*

caffeine, 22, 118
cake, angel food, 78
calcium, 66
calisthenics, 111
calories, 57, 58, 66, 104, 107-8, 109,
  111, 112
cancer, 105, 115, 116
carbohydrates, 59, 61
cardiovascular fitness, 105
cellulite: appearance, 16
  blood circulation, 30-1
  definition, 14-15
  diet and, 29-30
  ethnic and genetic variables, 28-9
  exercise and, 30
  lifecycle, 24-8
  psychological factors, 31
  structure, 18-19, *18*
  see also fat cells

chicken: chicken breasts Florentine,
  74
  dill chicken salad, 73
  lime-broiled chicken, 74
circulatory system, 21, 30-1, 116-17
climbing steps, 111, 112
clothes, 83
coffee granita, 78
coleslaw, 72
collagen, 65
connective tissue, 16, 18-19, *18*, 20,
  22, 65
contraceptive pill, 20, 26-7
cooking tips, 70

dancing, 111
desserts, 78
diaries, 121-5
diet, 29-30, 56-79
  alcohol, 66
  dining out, 66-7
  eating habits, 64-5
  fat content, 22, 26, 54, 57-9
  food combining, 64
  GREFLOF plan, 59-61, 68-70
  protein, 62-4
  questionnaire, 37-9
  recipes, 71-8
  sugar, 61-2
  vitamins and minerals, 65-6
dinner, 68
dip, super tofu spice, 73
doctors, 42-3

egg-white omelet, 71
Elevator Wait Lift, 89, *89*
endive salad, 72
endorphins, 107
energy requirements, 109
enzymes, 21-2
estrogen, 16, 20, 22, 25, 26, 28
ethnic variables, 28-9
exercise, 30, 80-113
  aerobic, 65, 81, 104-13
  Pressometrics, 81, 84-90
  questionnaire, 39-41
  Streamline Stretches, 81, 91-5
  Twelve-Minute Miracle, 81,
    96-103, 111
exfoliants, 117

fast food, 57, 67
fat cells: aerobic exercise, 105
  blood vessels, 21
  importance of, 16-18
  influence of hormones, 19-21
  liposuction, 44-6, *45*
  percentage of body weight, 44
  transport, storage and
    metabolism, 21-2, *23*
fats, in diet, 22, 26, 54, 57-9
fiber, 60-1, 63
fish, 63-4
fish oils, 58
Flamingo Stretch, 92, *92*
Flapper, 90, *90*
Floor Glider, 102, *102*
flounder in lettuce pouches, 75
food combining, 64
free radicals, 65
fructose, 59-60
fruit, 54, 59-61, *60*, 62, 69, 78

genetics, 28-9
glucocorticoids, 22
glycolysis, 105
goals, 49-50
golf, 111
grains, 63
GREFLOF plan, 54, 57, 64, 68-70
growth hormone, 22

habits, 52
Hand Heel Technique, massage,
  119, *119*
Happy Hundred, 103, *103*
Happy Hunger Helpers, 70
heart, aerobic exercise, 105
heart rate, *106*, 108
Hip Hugger, 85, *85*
honey, 62
hormones, 24
  contraceptive pills, 26-7
  effects on fat cells, 16, 19-21, 22
  pregnancy, 27
  puberty, 25-6
horseback riding, 111
hunger, 64, 107
hyaluronic acid, 26

insulin, 22, 59, 107

isometrics, 81, 84-90, 111

jogging, 110-12
joints, exercise, 91, 105

Kick 'em Out, 98, *98*
Kleinfelder's Syndrome, 20
Kneecap Kiss, 88, *88*
Knuckle Technique, massage, 119, *119*

lactic acid, 105
Latin Lover Leg Lift, 87, *87*
lemon-Dijon vinaigrette, 72
leotards, 83
lipids, 18
lipodysmorphia, 44
lipodystrophy, 15
lipolysis, 22
lipoprotein lipase, 21-2
liposuction, 44-6, *45*
liver, alcohol metabolism, 66
Low-High Spring, 99, *99*
lunch, 68
lymphatic system, 21, 115, 116

margarine, 58
massage, 115, 117-18, *119*
"mattress phenomenon", 16
measurements, *33*
meat, 64
medical examinations, 42-3
menopause, 27-8
metabolism, 21-2, 27, 105-6
Metronome, 101, *101*
minerals, 54, 65-6
monounsaturated fats, 58
muffins, apple bran, 71
muscles: aerobic exercise, 104-5
  metabolism, 106
  Pressometric exercises, 90
  stretching exercises, 91-5

nomograms, 44, 47

omelet, egg-white, 71
oral contraceptives, 20, 26-7
"orange peel phenomenon", 16, 19
osteoporosis, 28, 66
oxygen, aerobic exercise, 104-5
oxytocin, 22

pancakes, extra-light, 71
pasta primavera, 75
pear shape, 21
pears, blushing, 78
Pelvic Tuck, 85, *85*
pepper tricolore, 77
petrissage, 119
the Pill, 20, 26-7
pinch test, 16, *19*
pituitary hormones, 22
plaice in lettuce pouches, 75
polyunsaturated fats, 58
positive thinking, 51
posture, 31, 82-3, *82-3*
potato chips, fresh, 76
Power Palm Press, 90, *90*
pre-menstrual syndrome, 25
pregnancy, 27
Pressometrics, 81, 84-90
progesterone, 25, 26
prolactin, 22
protein, 54, 57, 62-4
puberty, 20, 25-6
pulse rate, *106*, 108

questionnaires, 32-41

ratatouille, 77
rebounding, 111, 113
recipes, 71-8
Reflection Reaction, 33, 107, 122
restaurants, 66-7
resting energy requirements, 109
rowing, 111
running, 110-12

Saddle Battle, 86, *86*
salads, 72-3
salmon salad, dill, 73
salt, 30, 59
sandwiches, 73
saturated fats, 58
sauce, super green spinach, 73
seafood on skewers, 74
Semaphore Wave, 103, *103*
shoes, 83
Sir Walter Raleigh, 92, *92*
skin brushing, 115, 116-17
skin cancer, 115, 116
skin care, 114-17
skipping ropes, 111, 112

snacks, 70
spinach: chicken breasts Florentine, 74
  spinach zucchini harmony, 77
  super green spinach sauce, 73
stairs, climbing, 112
Streamline Stretches, 81, 91-5
stretching exercises, 91-5
sugar, 54, 58-60, 61-2
sugar alcohols, 60
sun damage, skin, 115-16
sunscreens, 116
Superhero Lunge, 93, *93*
Suspended Animotion, 88, *88*
sweeteners, 54, 62
swimming, 111, 112-13

tai chi, 111
tanning, 115-16
tart vinaigrette, 72
tennis, 111
testosterone, 16, 20
theophyllin, 22, 118
Thigh High Back Kick, 100, *100*
Thigh High Side Stretch, 100, *100*
tofu spice dip, 73
triglycerides, 22
Turning Point, 49
turnips, terrific, 76
Twelve-Minute Miracle, 81, 96-103, 111

unsaturated fats, 58
UV radiation, 116

vegetables, 54, 59-61, *60*, 63, 69, 76-7
vinaigrettes, 72
visualization, 50-1, 53
vitamins, 54, 65, 69

walking, 104, 108-12
water retention, 20, 25, 26, 27, 28, 59
weight loss goals, 49-50
weight tables, 43, 47

yoga, 96, 111

zucchini spinach harmony, 77

■ Recommended reading

Cousins, Norman, *Anatomy of an Illness*: New York, W.W. Norton and Company, Inc., 1979.

Feldenkrais, Moshe, *Awareness Through Movement*: New York, Harper & Row, 1977.

Food and Nutrition Board, *Diet and Health Implications for Reducing Chronic Disease Risk*: National Research Council, Washington D.C.: National Academy Press, 1989.

Lalvani, Vimla, *Yogacise*: London, Hamlyn, 1994.

Netzer, Corinne T., *The Complete Book of Food Counts*: New York, Dell Publishing, 1988.

Ornish, Dean, *Eat More, Weigh Less. Dr. Dean Ornish's Life Choice Program for Losing Weight Safely While Eating Abundantly*: New York, Harper, 1994.

Pauling, Linus, *How to Live Longer and Feel Better*: New York, W.H. Freeman and Company, 1986.

Peale, Norman Vincent, *The Power of Positive Thinking*: Prentice Hall Inc., 1952.

Pinckney, Callan, *Callanetics*: New York, William Morrow and Company Inc.

Pritikin, N., and P.M., McGrady, *The Pritikin Program for Diet & Exercise*: New York, Grosset & Dunlap, 1979.

Restak, Richard, *The Brain Has a Mind of Its Own*: New York, Random House Inc., 1991.

Ronsard, Nicole, *Cellulite*: New York, Bantam Books, 1973.

Stehling, Wendy, *Thin Thighs in Thirty Days*: New York, Bantam Books, 1982 (revised 1989).

Walford, Roy L., *The 120 Year Diet: How to Double Your Vital Years*: New York: Simon and Schuster, 1986.

Walker, Norton and Frank, Angelo, *Rebounding Aerobics*: Edmonds, Washington: The National Institute of Reboundology and Health, Inc., 1981.

■ Author's acknowledgements

With very special thanks to my husband Peter and to Heather Nolan, Dina da Silva, Emilia Sequeira, Ruth Kava, Ph.D., Judith Stern, D.Sc., and Maxine Storch.

Author photograph on page iv by Manning Gurney.

■ Publisher's acknowledgements

The publisher would also like to thank Junckers, Wheaton Road, Witham, Essex CM8 3UJ, for the loan of the flooring used in the photographs in Chapter 8.